John W. Murphy, PhD, LCSW
John T. Pardeck, PhD
Editors

Disability Issues for Social Workers and Human Services Professionals in the Twenty-First Century

Disability Issues for Social Workers and Human Services Professionals in the Twenty-First Century has been co-published simultaneously as *Journal of Social Work in Disability & Rehabilitation*, Volume 4, Numbers 1/2 2005.

*Pre-publication
REVIEWS,
COMMENTARIES,
EVALUATIONS . . .*

"SOCIAL WORKERS AND HUMAN SERVICE PROFESSIONALS WILL FIND THIS MULTIDISCIPLINARY BOOK INFORMATIVE, PRACTICAL, AND INSPIRING. . . . A cutting-edge book for anyone who intends to effectively usher the field of disability into the twenty-first century. . . . Provides research-based and thought-provoking discussions on critical and emerging issues in the field of disability."

Francis K. Yuen, DSW, ACSW
*Professor, Division of Social Work
California State University
Sacramento*

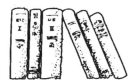

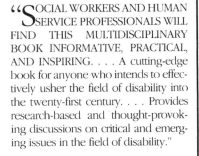

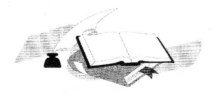

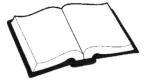

Disability Issues for Social Workers and Human Services Professionals in the Twenty-First Century

Disability Issues for Social Workers and Human Services Professionals in the Twenty-First Century has been co-published simultaneously as *Journal of Social Work in Disability & Rehabilitation,* Volume 4, Numbers 1/2 2005.

The *Journal of Social Work in Disability & Rehabilitation*™ Monographic "Separates"

Below is a list of "separates," which in serials librarianship means a special issue simultaneously published as a special journal issue or double-issue *and* as a "separate" hardbound monograph. (This is a format which we also call a "DocuSerial.")

"Separates" are published because specialized libraries or professionals may wish to purchase a specific thematic issue by itself in a format which can be separately cataloged and shelved, as opposed to purchasing the journal on an on-going basis. Faculty members may also more easily consider a "separate" for classroom adoption.

"Separates" are carefully classified separately with the major book jobbers so that the journal tie-in can be noted on new book order slips to avoid duplicate purchasing.

You may wish to visit Haworth's website at . . .

http://www.HaworthPress.com

. . . to search our online catalog for complete tables of contents of these separates and related publications.

You may also call 1-800-HAWORTH (outside US/Canada: 607-722-5857), or Fax 1-800-895-0582 (outside US/Canada: 607-771-0012), or e-mail at:

docdelivery@haworthpress.com

Disability Issues for Social Workers and Human Services Professionals in the Twenty-First Century

John W. Murphy
John T. Pardeck
Editors

Disability Issues for Social Workers and Human Services Professionals in the Twenty-First Century has been co-published simultaneously as *Journal of Social Work in Disability & Rehabilitation*, Volume 4, Numbers 1/2 2005.

The Haworth Social Work Practice Press
An Imprint of The Haworth Press, Inc.

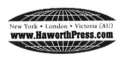

New York • London • Victoria (AU)
www.HaworthPress.com

Published by

The Haworth Social Work Practice Press®, 10 Alice Street, Binghamton, NY 13904-1580 USA

The Haworth Social Work Practice Press® is an imprint of The Haworth Press, Inc., 10 Alice Street, Binghamton, NY 13904-1580 USA.

Disability Issues for Social Workers and Human Services Professionals in the Twenty-First Century has been co-published simultaneously as *Journal of Social Work in Disability & Rehabilitation*™, Volume 4, Numbers 1/2 2005.

The development, preparation, and publication of this work has been undertaken with great care. However, the publisher, employees, editors, and agents of The Haworth Press and all imprints of The Haworth Press, Inc., including The Haworth Medical Press® and Pharmaceutical Products Press®, are not responsible for any errors contained herein or for consequences that may ensue from use of materials or information contained in this work. Opinions expressed by the author(s) are not necessarily those of The Haworth Press, Inc.

Cover design by Jennifer M. Gaska.

Library of Congress Cataloging-in-Publication Data

Disability issues for social workers and human services professionals in the twenty-first century/John W. Murphy guest editor, John T. Pardeck, editor
    p. cm.
        "Disability Issues for Social Workers and Human Services Professionals in the Twenty-First Century has been co-published simultaneously as Journal of Social Work in Disability & Rehabilitation, Volume 4, Numbers 1/2 2005."
        Includes bibliographical references and index.
      ISBN 0-7890-2713-5 (hard cover: alk. paper)–ISBN 0-7890-2714-3 (soft cover: alk. paper)
1. People with disabilities–Services for–United States. I. Murphy, John W. II. Pardeck, John T. III. Journal of social work in disability & rehabilitation.
HV1553.D5484 2005
362.4′0453--dc22   2004019284

Indexing, Abstracting & Website/Internet Coverage

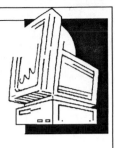

This section provides you with a list of major indexing & abstracting services and other tools for bibliographic access. That is to say, each service began covering this periodical during the year noted in the right column. Most Websites which are listed below have indicated that they will either post, disseminate, compile, archive, cite or alert their own Website users with research-based content from this work. (This list is as current as the copyright date of this publication.)

Abstracting, Website/Indexing Coverage . . . . Year When Coverage Began

- *CINAHL (Cumulative Index to Nursing & Allied Health Literature), in print, EBSCO, and SilverPlatter, DataStar, and PaperChase. (Support materials include Subject Heading List, Database Search Guide, and instructional video).*
  <http://www.cinahl.com> 2003
- *e-psyche, LLC <http://www.e-psyche.net>* 2002
- *EBSCOhost Electronic Journals Service (EJS)*
  <http://ejournals.ebsco.com> 2002
- *Exceptional Child Education Resources (ECER), (CD/ROM from SilverPlatter and hard copy)*
  <http://www.ericec.org/ecer-db.html> 2003
- *Family & Society Studies Worldwide <http://www.nisc.com>* 2002
- *Family Index Database <http://www.familyscholar.com>* 2003
- *Google <http://www.google.com>* 2004
- *Google Scholar <http://scholar.google.com>* 2004
- *Haworth Document Delivery Center* 2002
- *Higher Education Abstracts, providing the latest in research & theory in more than 140 major topics* 2003
- *IBZ International Bibliography of Periodical Literature*
  <http://www.saur.de> 2002

(continued)

Special Bibliographic Notes related to special journal issues (separates) and indexing/abstracting:

- indexing/abstracting services in this list will also cover material in any "separate" that is co-published simultaneously with Haworth's special thematic journal issue or DocuSerial. Indexing/abstracting usually covers material at the article/chapter level.
- monographic co-editions are intended for either non-subscribers or libraries which intend to purchase a second copy for their circulating collections.
- monographic co-editions are reported to all jobbers/wholesalers/approval plans. The source journal is listed as the "series" to assist the prevention of duplicate purchasing in the same manner utilized for books-in-series.
- to facilitate user/access services all indexing/abstracting services are encouraged to utilize the co-indexing entry note indicated at the bottom of the first page of each article/chapter/contribution.
- this is intended to assist a library user of any reference tool (whether print, electronic, online, or CD-ROM) to locate the monographic version if the library has purchased this version but not a subscription to the source journal.
- individual articles/chapters in any Haworth publication are also available through the Haworth Document Delivery Service (HDDS).

Disability Issues for Social Workers and Human Services Professionals in the Twenty-First Century

CONTENTS

In Memoriam

John T. Pardeck died on November 6, 2004 after a year and a half bout with cancer. He was a scholar, social activist, and a friend to many persons. Additionally, he was the founding editor of this journal. This review owes its inspiration and direction to his tireless efforts. In this regard, he believed that a place is needed where scholarship could be presented that would eventually lead to improving the lives of the disabled. He felt strongly that these persons constituted a minority group that is denied rights that most persons take for granted. His regular contributions to the *Journal of Social Work in Disability & Rehabilitation* and other scholarly venues will be missed, along with his sense of humor and friendship.

ABOUT THE EDITORS

John W. Murphy received his PhD degree in 1981 from Ohio State University. His interests are sociological theory, social philosophy, and globalization. He has published books related to the community mental health movement, the computerization of social service agencies, and contemporary social theory. His most recent books are: *Postmodernism, Unraveling Racism, and Democratic Institutions,* 1997 (w/Jung Choi), *Computers, Human Interaction, and Organizations,* 2001 (w/ Vicente Berdayes), and *Communication and Social Action Research*, 2001 (w/several co-authors). Most recently he has published articles such as *Reply to Ulmer: Symbolic Interactionism or a Structural Alternative* (w/ Luigi Esposito), *Gregorio Morales: Etica y Estetica Cuantica* (w/ Manolo Caro), *Another Step in the Study of Race Relations* (w/Luigi Esposito), and *Does Postmodernism Undermine Politics?*

John T. Pardeck, PhD, was formerly Professor of Social Work in the School at Southwest Missouri State University. Prior to this position, he was Chair of the Department of Social Work at Southeast Missouri State University. He was an advocate for persons with disabilities and for interpreting the Americans With Disabilities Act to both private and public sector organizations.

Dr. Pardeck was the author of *Social Work After the Americans With Disabilities Act: New Challenges and Opportunities for Social Services Professionals.* He has published numerous articles on disabilities and related topics. His publications have appeared in journals that include *Social Work, Child Welfare, Families in Society,* and *Research on Social Work Practice.* He has published over 100 articles in professional and academic journals and has authored, co-authored, edited, or co-edited over a dozen books, including *Social Work: Seeking Relevancy in the Twenty-First Century, Using*

Books in Clinical Social Work Practice, Reason and Rationality in Health and Human Services Delivery, and *Postmodernism, Religion, and the Future of Social Work* (all published by The Haworth Press, Inc.). Dr. Pardeck served on the boards of several statewide social service organizations as well as on the editorial boards of several national and international journals.

About the Contributors

Carol J. Evans, PhD, Director, Child & Family Mental Health Services Division, trained in community psychology at the University of Missouri-Kansas City. Dr. Evans has been principal investigator of the Starting Early, Starting Smart grant, a project that linked very young children and their families from a pediatric setting to mental health and other resources in the community. Her current projects include the evaluation of School-based Prevention Intervention and Resources IniTiative (SPIRIT), a substance abuse prevention project funded by the Division of Alcohol and Drug Abuse, Missouri Department of Mental Health. Dr. Evan's research interests include consumer involvement, children's mental health issues and mental health service systems research.

Paula Gilbert, MA, MSW, LCSW, is Assistant Professor and Director of Psychological Services at Bronx Community College of the City University of New York. She has studied and worked with adults with Attention Deficit Hyperactivity Disorder in mental health and college settings over the last ten years. Professor Gilbert can be reached at Bronx Community College, Psychological Services, Loew Hall, University Avenue and West 181st Street, Bronx, NY 10453, (718) 289-5873 or e-mail: paula.gilbert@bcc.cuny.edu

Diane L. Green received her PhD in Social Work from the University of Texas at Austin and her MSW from the University of Central Florida. Dr. Green's practice experience includes administration, direct services in group homes for foster care, juvenile delinquents, hospice, and a Child/Adolescent Psychiatric Hospital. Her research and scholarly interests include stress and coping, grief and loss, end-of-life issues, and HIV/AIDS.

Michele Hawkins earned her MSW from the University of Missouri and her PhD in Public Health Education from Southern Illinois University. She is a licensed clinical social worker and a member of the Academy of Certified Social Workers, the Baccalaureate Social Work Program Directors, National Association Social Work and Council on Social Work Education. She has published articles in the areas of mental health and education, child welfare and health, and social policy.

Wesley Hawkins earned his MSW from Catholic University, Washington, DC. His PhD is in Public Health Education from Southern Illinois University. Previously, Dr. Hawkins was on faculty at the Johns Hopkins University and the University of Oregon. Most recently, he directed psycho-social interventions in the Clinical Trials Division of the National Institute of Drug Abuse. Dr. Hawkins has numerous publications and grant funding in his research areas of adolescent depression and drug abuse. He presently serves on the Editorial Board, Book Review Editor, and as a reviewer for *Children and Youth Services.*

Virginia Rondero Hernandez is Assistant Professor in the Department of Social Work Education, California State University, Fresno. She also serves as the Associate Director of the Central California Children's Institute at the CSU-Fresno Campus where she provides leadership and oversight of funded research in the areas of children's health and welfare. Dr. Rondero Hernandez earned her MSW from California State University, Sacramento and her PhD from the Mandel School of Applied Social Sciences at Case Western Reserve University. Prior to accepting her post in California, she taught at Texas State University, San Marcos, TX and Our Lady of the Lake University in San Antonio, TX. Her research interests include children's health, developmental disabilities, and juvenile justice.

John Q. Hodges is Assistant Professor of Social Work at the University of Missouri, Columbia. His research interests include mental health consumer-run services, consumer perspectives on the mental health service system, innovations in mental health care service delivery, and severe mental illness. He received his PhD from the University of California, Berkeley School of Social Welfare.

Jennifer Mallow is a school social worker with Communities-in-Schools in Hays County, TX. She holds an MSW from Texas State University-San Marcos. Her research interests include school social work, disabilities, and children's mental health. She was a graduate student intern during the project described in the article.

Martha Markward earned her MSW and PhD in Education from the University of Illinois, Urbana-Champaign and has practice experience as a school social worker. She is Associate Professor in the University of Missouri's School of Social Work in Columbia where she teaches across the curriculum at the graduate level. Most recently, she has taught research, advanced policy analysis with families and children, and evaluation of clinical practice. Dr. Markward's research and scholarly publications focus on topics related to the mental health of families and children. Currently, Dr. Markward is co-evaluating a gender-specific violence prevention project being implemented with preteen girls in inner-city St. Louis.

Debra J. Morrison-Ortin is Assistant Professor at California State University, Bakersfield. She has earned an MSW from George Warren Brown School of Social Work and her PhD from the University of Texas at Austin in Special Education and Rehabilitation. Her research interests include substance abuse, family violence, health and mental health issues, and social work education.

Katherine Selber is Associate Professor at the School of Social Work, Texas State University-San Marcos. Dr. Selber holds an MSSW form the University of Houston and a PhD degree from the University of Texas-Austin. Prior to completing her doctoral degree and joining the faculty in 1997, she was a Field Director and clinical faculty member at the University of Texas-Austin for twelve years. She also taught at the National Autonomous University of Mexico in Mexico City where she held a joint appointment as a researcher at their National Institute of Psychiatry. Her research interests include disabilities, criminal justice, and social work education.

Mary Tijerina is Assistant Professor and Director of the BSW program in the School of Social Work at Texas State University-San Marcos. Dr. Tijerina holds MSSW and PhD degrees from the University of Texas at Austin. Prior to joining the faculty in 2001, she was a grant coordinator for the Public Health Leadership in Genetics project funded by the Texas Department of Health. She also served as a research associate in the Division of Student Affairs at Texas State and as Director of Program Services for the Texas Commission on Alcohol and Drug Abuse. Her research interests include health and illness, substance abuse, and social work education.

Dong Pil Yoon, PhD, is Assistant Professor at the School of Social Work, University of Missouri-Columbia. He has taught advanced social policy for planning and administration, organization theory, social welfare history, and quantitative research methods. He has conducted a number of studies on intercountry adoption, religiousness/spirituality, and rural social work. In 2004, two articles entitled *"Intercountry Adoption: The Importance of Ethnic Socialization and Subjective Well-Being for Korean-Born Adopted Children"* and *"Religiousness/Spirituality and Subjective Well-Being Among Rural Elderly Whites, African Americans, and Native Americans"* were published in *Journal of Ethnic & Cultural Diversity in Social Work* and *Journal of Human Behavior in the Social Environment*, respectively.

Preface

Three dominant models have emerged for understanding the meaning of disability; these include the moral, medical and minority models. Each of these models views disability from a unique and very different perspective. In the twentieth century the moral and medical models dominated the worldviews of most people concerning how a disability was understood and viewed (Pardeck, 1998).

The moral model offers the oldest understanding of disability and is found in many cultures (Olkin, 1999). In Native American and Asian cultures, the model views a disability as being out of the natural order of things (Longmore, 1987). The basic tenets of the moral model can also be found in Judeo-Christian thought as well as in other religions. In the Judeo-Christian tradition, the moral model suggests that a disability is seen as "divine retribution" (Florion, 1982). Given this tradition, the person with a disability may feel shame and the family with a child with a disability, for example, may feel they are being punished for some kind of moral failure.

Throughout the twentieth century, the medical model influenced society's understanding of disability. This model attributes pathology to a biological and molecular basis. It divides the mind and body into separate parts; this division has its roots in Dualism, a perspective formulated by Descartes (Pardeck and Yuen, 1999). The medical model argues that a disability is a medical problem, a defect or failure of a body system denoting abnormality and pathology (Smart, 2001). It is based on the assumption that there is a cure for disabilities; science simply must discover those cures. As a model of disability, it has a tendency to not consider the impact of the environment on the person. That is, the disability is within the person; the person must thus adapt to his or her

[Haworth co-indexing entry note]: "Preface." Murphy, John W., and John T. Pardeck. Co-published simultaneously in *Journal of Social Work in Disability & Rehabilitation* (The Haworth Social Work Practice Press, an imprint of The Haworth Press, Inc.) Vol. 4, No. 1/2, 2005, pp. xxi-xxiii; and: *Disability Issues for Social Workers and Human Services Professionals in the Twenty-First Century* (ed: John W. Murphy, and John T. Pardeck) The Haworth Social Work Practice Press, an imprint of The Haworth Press, Inc., 2005, pp. xvii-xix. Single or multiple copies of this article are available for a fee from The Haworth Document Delivery Service [1-800-HAWORTH, 9:00 a.m. - 5:00 p.m. (EST). E-mail address: docdelivery@haworthpress.com].

xvii

environment. Engel (1977, p. 130) concludes that the medical model is "the dominant folk model of disease in the western world."

The most recent model to emerge, the minority model, views a disability as being a social construct that lies in the environment and not the person. This model sees persons with disabilities as a minority–in the same way that persons of color are a minority–that have been denied their civil rights, equal access, and legal protections (Smart, 2001). Like other minorities, people with disabilities are confronted with prejudice and discrimination, social isolation, unequal treatment, economic dependency, and high rates of unemployment (Biklen, 1988; Florian, 1982). An objective of the minority model is to empower persons with disabilities so that they might change the social, physical, and political barriers that have oppressed them.

This book is based on the assumption that the moral model of disability is dated. If anything, it is based on superstition and ignorance. Within the professions that work with people with disabilities, there is simply no place for such a view. The medical model dominated the field of disability in the twentieth century. The entire social services delivery system continues to be based on this model. This domination is not only for medical purposes but includes a hidden political agenda, that being there are many vested interests to be served. For example, home based care is much less expensive than nursing home care for those with disabilities. However, if people with disabilities were moved from nursing homes to home based care a great deal of money would be lost by the nursing home industry. The disability rights movement has challenged the basic assumptions of the medical model. The goal of this movement is to move the helping professions toward the newer minority model.

This book is based on the view that the minority model of disability is emerging as the dominant model for understanding disability in the twenty-first century. For example, the Americans With Disabilities Act (ADA) is grounded in the minority model. This book offers a complete analysis of the ADA. There is also a chapter on changing norms and disability that will help the reader gain insight into why the meaning of disability continues to change over time. This chapter also illustrates why a disability is a social construct and not necessarily something that is inherent to the person. The social problems related to the medical model are also offered in the work. These include the medication of children with disabilities and the problems created by managed care. The challenges of new ideas emerging in the helping professions are also covered. These include the role of spirituality and religion in treating those with disabilities and the new view that a disability should be seen as a part of cultural diversity just like race and religion are currently viewed. Many of the chapters offer groundbreaking material that has not been discussed in the social work or human services literature on disability.

The goal of this book is to cover new areas of disability that have not been covered in the social work literature. It is designed for practitioners and social work academics for use in the classroom. It attempts to move the reader in a direction that legitimates the minority model and to help practitioners think about the meaning of disability in new ways in the twenty-first century.

John W. Murphy
John T. Pardeck
Editors

REFERENCES

Biklen, D. (1988). The myth of clinical judgment. *Journal of Social Issues*, 44, 127-140.

Engel, G. L. (1977). The need for a new medical model: A challenge for biomedicine. *Science*, 196, 129-136.

Florian, V. (1982). Cross-cultural differences in attitudes towards disabled persons: A study of Jewish and Arab youth in Israel. *International Journal of Intercultural Relations*, 6, 291-299.

Longmore, P. K. (1987). Uncovering the hidden history of people with disabilities. *Review in American History*, 15, 355-364.

Olkin, R. (1999). The personal, professional and political: When clients have disabilities. In E. Kaschak and M. Hill (Eds.), *Beyond the rule book: Moral issues and dilemmas in the practice of psychotherapy* (pp. 87-103). New York: The Haworth Press, Inc.

Pardeck, J. T. (1998). *Social work after the Americans With Disabilities Act: New challenges and opportunities for social service professionals*. Westport, CT: Auburn House.

Pardeck, J. T., & Yuen, K. O. (Eds.) (1999). *Family health: A holistic approach to social work practice*. Westport, CT: Auburn House.

Smart, J. (2001). *Disability, society, and the individual*. Gaithersburg, MD: Aspen Publishers, Inc.

Introduction

John W. Murphy
John T. Pardeck

This volume explores topics critical to the field of disability in the 21st century. These topics are examined at the practice, policy and program, and theoretical levels. Issues explored include the role of religion and spirituality in the rehabilitation process; the use of medication in treating disability; Attention-Deficit/Hyperactivity Disorder in college students; cultural diversity and disability; civil rights of persons with disabilities; computer technology and disability; and managed mental health care and disability. Two decades ago these issues were not even mentioned in the field of disability; in the 21st century, they have emerged as critical topics, particularly in the fields of social work and the human services.

SECTION I.
DISABILITY PRACTICE
IN THE TWENTY-FIRST CENTURY

The first paper in this issue presents a study on the use of religion and spiritual strategies in the rehabilitation process. The research found that

[Haworth co-indexing entry note]: "Introduction." Murphy, John W., and John T. Pardeck. Co-published simultaneously in *Journal of Social Work in Disability & Rehabilitation* (The Haworth Social Work Practice Press, an imprint of The Haworth Press, Inc.) Vol. 4, No. 1/2, 2005, pp. 1-4; and: *Disability Issues for Social Workers and Human Services Professionals in the Twenty-First Century* (ed: John W. Murphy, and John T. Pardeck) The Haworth Social Work Practice Press, an imprint of The Haworth Press, Inc., 2005, pp. 1-4. Single or multiple copies of this article are available for a fee from The Haworth Document Delivery Service [1-800-HAWORTH, 9:00 a.m. - 5:00 p.m. (EST). E-mail address: docdelivery@haworthpress.com].

http://www.haworthpress.com/web/JSWDR
Digital Object Identifier: 10.1300/J198v04n01_01

religion and spirituality are thought to be critical to treating persons with disabilities; however, there is a real problem in defining what religion and spirituality mean in terms of clinical practice. The use of religion and spirituality are outside the traditional medical model approach to rehabilitation; thus it is difficult to convince those in mainstream medicine to accept the importance of these issues when working with patients.

The paper on medication focuses on children in foster care. Many children in foster care are confronted with a number of disabilities, particularly emotional and behavioral disabilities. The research conducted in this paper reports a large percentage of children in foster care receive medication as a strategy to control the effects of their disability. As has been the tradition in medicine, it is much less expensive to use medication versus using other kinds of therapies to treat disabilities. The result of this approach is that entirely too many children in placement receive medication when other more expensive approaches such as family therapy would be more effective for the children and their families. There is little to suggest that the over-medication of children not only in foster care but also the larger society will change in the near future.

Attention-Deficit/Hyperactivity Disorder has emerged as a legitimate disability among adults. For a number of years it was thought that only children were the likely candidates for this disability. The paper on this topic reviews the literature on the topic of Attention-Deficit/Hyperactivity Disorder in adults and then explores how it impacts college students as a disability requiring academic accommodations. As would be suspected it is very difficult to convince institutions of higher learning to accept this notion.

The final paper in the practice section of the issue explores the concept of disability as part of the larger notion of cultural diversity. Considering disability as part of cultural diversity has only been accepted by a limited number of social work professionals; most social work programs only view cultural diversity including the traditional notions of race, ethnicity and religion. What is unique about this paper is it suggests children's books can be an extremely effective approach for teaching other nondisabled children about children with various disabilities. The same strategy can also be used to teach adults about people with disabilities. In essence, this paper presents two new ideas to the field of disability: disability and cultural diversity, and the use of literature for understanding the problems facing persons with disabilities.

SECTION II.
DISABILITY POLICY AND PROGRAMS
IN THE TWENTY-FIRST CENTURY

The first paper in this section explores the use of computer technology, specifically the Internet, in providing help to families and others about children with disabilities. The paper conducts research on how an effective website is created and maintained on the topic of disability. Those participating in the study report that websites can be a very effective tool for understanding disability and those websites provide much important information for parents and others for providing help for children with disabilities.

The second paper in this section deals with mental health consumers and managed care. The general problems of medical services delivered through managed care have been widely known for a number of years. Mental health services and managed care has only emerged as a critical issue over the last several years. This paper explores those issues.

The final paper explores civil rights and persons with disabilities. The emphasis in the paper is on the Americans With Disabilities Act (ADA). The ADA was signed into law in 1990. Advocates in the field of disabilities, and obviously persons with disabilities, felt that the new law would have a profound effect on ending discrimination against persons with disabilities. What the paper clearly illustrates is that the United States Supreme Court has greatly limited the impact of the ADA and that there has been a great deal of concern among disability rights activists about the limitations placed on the ADA by the Court. Even though the Court has limited the impact of the ADA, a number of federal agencies have been aggressive in their enforcement of the ADA. The paper concludes that what is most important at this time is to use advocacy as a tool for ensuring civil rights for persons with disabilities and as a strategy for convincing the United States Congress to restore the damage that has been done to the ADA by the United States Supreme Court.

SECTION III.
DISABILITY THEORY
IN THE TWENTY-FIRST CENTURY

The paper in this section discusses how and why the norms for defining disability continue to change. This analysis illustrates the social nature of a disability and that the changing norms for treating disability are a result of the social construction process. This analysis is grounded in a postmodern analysis, a notion that has only entered the field of disability in the 21st century.

CONCLUSION

The topics covered in this collection cover emerging topics in the field of disability in the 21st century. Many of these topics are only now being discussed as critical to the field of disability. Many of them are particularly important to the field of social work and the human services in general. For example, computer technology through the use of the Internet has been found to be a very effective tool for providing resources to persons with disabilities; this new revelation has not been widely accepted by social work or the human services. The topic of religion and spirituality as part of the treatment process is not widely accepted among practitioners even though they are important notions to clients. The civil rights of persons with disabilities is not well understood by social workers; furthermore, limited content is taught on this topic in social work programs. Human service agencies have a tendency to reject civil rights for persons with disabilities.

In conclusion, the emerging disabilities issues in the 21st century will become mainstream topics as time passes. The goal of this issue is to push the field of disability to begin considering the importance of these topics. It is particularly critical for social workers and human services workers to understand their importance to persons with disabilities.

SECTION I
DISABILITY PRACTICE
IN THE TWENTY-FIRST CENTURY

The Use of Religion
and Spiritual Strategies
in Rehabilitation

Debra J. Morrison-Orton

SUMMARY. Recently the helping professions have reopened the debate about utilizing religion or spirituality in both education and practice. In this study, in-depth interviews were completed to identify what, if any, strategies rehabilitation professionals had utilized in practice. Four major themes evolved from participants: (1) denial of having used strategies; (2) use of the concepts for their own benefit;

Debra J. Morrison-Orton, PhD, LMSW-ACP, is Assistant Professor, Department of Social Work, California State University, Bakersfield, CA.

[Haworth co-indexing entry note]: "The Use of Religion and Spiritual Strategies in Rehabilitation." Orton-Morrison, Debra J. Co-published simultaneously in *Journal of Social Work in Disability & Rehabilitation* (The Haworth Social Work Practice Press, an imprint of The Haworth Press, Inc.) Vol. 4, No. 1/2, 2005, pp. 5-41; and: *Disability Issues for Social Workers and Human Services Professionals in the Twenty-First Century* (ed: John W. Murphy, and John T. Pardeck) The Haworth Social Work Practice Press, an imprint of The Haworth Press, Inc., 2005, pp. 5-41. Single or multiple copies of this article are available for a fee from The Haworth Document Delivery Service [1-800-HAWORTH, 9:00 a.m. - 5:00 p.m. (EST). E-mail address: docdelivery@haworthpress.com].

(3) use of the concepts for client benefit; and (4) the use of multiple religious or spiritual strategies. Implications for professional and continuing education are addressed. Lastly, suggestions for future research are highlighted. *[Article copies available for a fee from The Haworth Document Delivery Service: 1-800-HAWORTH. E-mail address: <docdelivery@ haworthpress.com> Website: <http://www.HaworthPress.com> © 2005 by The Haworth Press, Inc. All rights reserved.]*

KEYWORDS. Use of spirituality and religion, rehabilitation, social work, health, disabilities, training, education

INTRODUCTION

While the process of rehabilitation is broad and varies by setting and discipline, Byrd (1999) made the point that rehabilitation should consider the whole person. He noted that professionals utilize the bio-psycho-social model in assessing and treating clients, but he argued that it is critical to incorporate the spiritual and religious elements of an individual's life into the helping process. Although there is a call to include spirituality and or religion into the helping professions there are no clear guidelines about what spiritual (or religion) means or what one does to "concern one's self directly with . . . spirit" (Byrd, 1999). Nor does Byrd identify what he meant by "reliance upon their spiritual resources" in the practice setting. An earlier study (Morrison-Orton, in press) strove to define the concepts of spirituality and religion as conceived by rehabilitation professionals. The remaining issue is once a particular understanding is developed, how do rehabilitation workers apply or mobilize spiritual or religious concepts in a rehabilitation practice?

Literature Review

Of all the human dimensions, spirituality has enjoyed only limited sporadic episodes of study. Scientists, it seems, prefer to leave most of the research to clergy, clerics, and mystics (Barbour, 1997). The issues surrounding the application of spiritual and religious concepts to daily living and dying have had a long history in the United States. The role these concepts have had on public life began in early and had many of its roots following the same trajectory as those seen in the fallout from the English Elizabethan Poor Laws (1601). These laws often reinforced dominant social values that were institutionalized via the volunteer work of church or religious communities and organizations. While some of these social values (Holland, 1989; Reid & Popple, 1992) included teaching 'right' moral behaviors others pertained to alms or charity (Lindberg, 1993; Van Wormer, 1997), compassion (Olasky, 1992), and caring (Brabeck, 1989; Dunajski, 1994). Society tried to figure out what to do with individuals who did not fit the norm of mainstream society physically, emotionally, socially, religiously, sexually, or racially (Axinn & Levin, 1997; Wuthnow & Hodgkinson, 1990). It became apparent those who could not be woven smoothly into the dominant social fabric would not disappear but had to be dealt with or provided for or protected (Skopal, 1995; Trattner, 1994). The call to consider the incorporation of spiritual or religious concepts into the rehabilitation practice has grown louder. Today, President George W. Bush has called on faith-based organizations to take over and or enhance social services more recently supported by the government.

The focus of this research centers on the concepts of religion and spirituality as rehabilitation professionals apply these concepts when intervening with persons experiencing physical, cognitive and or mental health disabilities, or their loved ones and or caregivers. The way any person believes, the manner in which a person's culture ascribes meaning to behaviors, language, and rituals will all impact an individual's values and worldview. Clients and rehabilitation professionals will share in this co-created reality. This reality will, in turn, affect mental and physical health of clients (Pellebon & Anderson, 1999) and impact the way professionals interact with clients.

Spirituality and Religion:
Their Relationship to Health, Disability and Adjustment

Serving individuals with disabilities presents many opportunities for rehabilitation professionals to come face to face with spiritual and religious issues. Many professionals have spoken directly to the issues (Havranek, 1999; Canda, 1995). McCarthy (1995b) postulated that while the general population has the commonality of religiosity

> there is likely to be an increase, within the rehabilitation target population, in spiritual interests or needs associated with the fact that many clients seek or are referred to counseling because they are confronting personal crises. Such situations tend to stimulate contemplation of life's meaning or to test their faith. (p. 189)

Hunt (1996) stated that in working with individuals infected with HIV, rehabilitation professionals should not "shy away from discussing . . . issues related to religion and spirituality . . ." (p. 71). Keith Byrd (1999) suggested, "the greatest potential for healing from a spiritual frame of reference can be found in a relationship between the person with a disability or chronic illness and God" (p. 12). Carolyn Vash (1981) contrasted the experience of having a disability in a spiritual sense and a technological sense. She called for the integration of the concept of transcendence into a stage model for integrating a disability into one's life. Conrad (1989) also believed spirituality was a potentially positive and helpful tool in the taming of the harsh and often seemingly inhumane application of biomedical ethics faced in the bureaucratic organization. O'Hanlon's (1999) suggestion to use the arts to connect to self and others also may be one step in humanizing impersonal or sterile bureaucratic health and justice systems caring for people.

Modern psychoneuroimmunologists believe the spiritual dimension of an individual has its organic and physical correlates in the essential organization of genetics (Jerotic, 1997; Trieschmann, 1995). Introducing the spiritual principle into the treatment of mentally ill patients can help restore the physical-mental-spiritual balance of the individual. Jerotic (1998) called for the introduction of the spiritual principle within group therapy with its main purpose being to strengthen Victor Frankl's concept of the "will to" or for meaning (1969, 1986). This according to Jerotic helps to strengthen an individual's psychoneuroimmunological organization.

The medical model assumes that good physical health produces happiness and well-being and the focus of rehabilitation efforts is the happiness of the individual with a disability (Trieschmann, 1995). Trieschmann believes that rehabilitation has always emphasized the whole person, including the emotions of the individual and their environments. She encouraged rehabilitation professionals to consider psycho neuroimmunology as closer to the whole person model of intervention. Specifically she argued for an energy model, which integrates "the body, mind, emotions, and soul into a philosophy of health and wellness which returns humanity to a linkage with nature" (p. 222). She linked this model to the field of physics where energy cannot be destroyed but is interdependent and transformed. Using an oriental philosophy and strategies to create spiritual harmony and tranquility she identified a goal of addressing these spiritual issues as a way "to provide a methodology that allows us to live more comfortably with 'what is' . . . so we do not burn ourselves up with sustained emotional reactions . . ." (p. 226).

Multiple articles have appeared in the literature describing how individuals with disabilities or their caregivers have found spiritual or religious interventions important to the process of living with, adjusting to, or working with those with disabilities (Dunbar, Mueller, Medina, & Wolf, 1998; Kaplan, Marks, & Mertens, 1997; Lane, 1992, 1995; Rotteveel, 1999).

Sistler and Washington (1999) found that in a caregiver group that focused on the serenity prayer and participant spirituality, African American women perceived a greater sense of control, greater confidence in their ability to problem solve, and achieved a greater sense of happiness and well-being when caring for a parent with dementia. Caregivers of Alzheimer patients who regularly worshiped and reported that their spiritual needs were being met had greater well-being and decreased stress than those caregivers who reported that their spiritual needs are not being adequately addressed (Burgener, 1994). In elder patients living in nursing homes there was a reverse relationship between worship practices and functional and perceived disability (Idler & Kasal, 1997a, 1997b).

Anderson, Anderson, and Felsenthal (1993) surveyed individuals released from a rehabilitation hospital and discovered that 45% did not believe enough attention was given to their spiritual needs while hospitalized. Among cancer patients being treated in a hospice setting, stronger religious beliefs were associated with reduced anxiety (Kaczoroswki, 1989). Patients with chronic medical illnesses, such as cystic fibrosis (Stern et al., 1992), cancer (Smith, Stefanek, Joseph, & Verdieck, 1993), lung cancer (Ginsburg et al., 1995), diabetes (Landis, 1996) and chronic renal failure (O'Brien, 1982) frequently used religious and spiritual adjuncts to medical care and reported positive benefits from these practices. Yates et al. (1981) found cancer patients and their religious beliefs were associated with reduced levels of pain. Additionally, Comstock and Partridge (1972) found a relationship between regular (weekly) church attendance and significantly lower rates of coronary disease, emphysema, cirrhosis, and suicide. A study of heart transplant patients revealed that religious beliefs and practices at the time of the transplant predicted improved physical, functioning, adherence to medical regiments, higher self esteem, and diminished anxiety about health one year post surgery (Harris et al., 1995).

In serving clients who had severe mental illness Garske (1999) emphasized the importance of the relationship the client had with self and others in the form of social support and community to help maximize the potential of these individuals. It was argued that community and social support might come from involvement in faith communities (Peck, 1993; Sullivan, 1992). Other elements identified with religion and spirituality include Carl Rogers' (1942) expectations for empathy, unconditional positive regard, and congruence; inclusion (Atkins, 1988; Sullivan, 1992); community (O'Hanlon, 1999; Peck, 1993); and relationship to self and others (Taylor & Wolfer, 1999). Several authors have called for the inclusion of spirituality in mental health service delivery to include putting the 'soul' back in psychotherapy (Becvar, 1997; Cornett, 1998; Goldberg, 1996; Haake, 1996; Pezzulo, 1997; Sheridan, 1995; Simons, 1992). Some mental health patients in one study identified sin as a reason for their mental illness (Sheehan & Kroll, 1990). In a cross-sectional survey with a case-control design for the study sub-sample, 720 patients were reinterviewed from a previously large-scale community study of psychiatric epidemiology. The authors of another study concluded patients with suicidal feelings are more likely to be female, to have been treated for other psychiatric symptoms (especially depression) and medical symptoms, to be socially isolated, to have fewer religious affiliations, less religious attendance and prayer, and have a greater frequency of stressful life events than patients who were not suicidal (Paykel, Myers, Lindenthal, & Tanner, 1974). Others have looked at spirituality in treating clients with depression (Cadwallander, 1991; Kaiser-Ryan, 1991), severe mental illness (Sullivan, 1992), including schizophrenia (Walsh, 1995), and multiple personality disorder (Iorfido, 1996). Data gathered from 131 community-dwelling chronically ill elderly revealed significant findings of a correlation between mental health, coping with pain of chronic illness and "closeness to God" (Burke, 1999).

Substance abuse rehabilitation has a long history of using spirituality in the healing process of traditional self-help groups (Gregoire, 1995; Krill, 1990b; Morell, 1996). These programs build in components of what has been described as spirituality. The components include respect for self and others, dignity for all, compassion, belief in a higher power, forgiveness, and service to others. AA forbids endorsement of any religious or political organization, including religious organizations. The traditional philosophy and governing rules of AA makes an important distinction between spirituality and religion stating that there is no requirement to believe in a particular God, but rather a higher power of the individual's choice. Data suggests that persons in recovery who embrace a higher power often undergo life-altering transformations

(Green, Fullilove, & Fullilove, 1998), which can contribute to long-term abstinence and recovery. There are studies linking religious affiliation that seem to have a moderating effect on an individual's behavior of alcohol and drugs use (Burkett, 1977; Dudley, Mutch, & Cruise, 1987). Miller (1998) believed that religious involvement and spiritual re-engagement during recovery was correlated with recovery and abstinence.

Other rehabilitation workers who have acquired disabilities themselves have written about the importance of spirituality in their healing. One example is the story of Megel Elie (1995), a graduate of Tulane Medical School. Shortly after graduation at age 27, Elie had a sickle cell attack that left her in a coma for 41 days. When she regained consciousness she expected to get up and walk. However, her ability to do anything for herself was gone. After many losing struggles to return to her premorbid state she came to realize that God had always been the one who had given her success. She believed that when she realized this she was finally able to return to a part-time medical career. She believed her return was a direct result of divine intervention and that she must not lose sight of whom and what brought her to this less self-centered point of view and a meaningful life.

Purpose of the Study

Quantitative strategies have been inadequate in capturing these intangible concepts. Additionally the use of quantitative methods have not revealed the details of how rehabilitation professionals have utilized spiritual or religious strategies in practice (Larsen & Larsen, 1994; Matthews & Saunders, 1997). This study utilized phenomenology to address these issues by asking individual rehabilitation professionals if they incorporated spiritual or religious strategies in their professional practices and if so what were they. Probes were used. These were questions associated with if, when and or how do they apply the concepts in practice. The respondents were also encouraged to discuss why they choose not to use religion or spirituality in practice. It was inevitable that personal spiritual or religious orientations presented themselves during the interviews. Participants were afforded the opportunity to discuss the impact these personal beliefs had on their lives and professional practice. The reader is encouraged to draw their own conclusions about how these views may have influenced the individual rehabilitation professional's practice.

METHODOLOGY

According to Patton (1990) the central question asked by phenomenological research is "What is the structure and essence of experience of this phenomenon for these people?" (p. 88). The goal of the phenomenological method is to ascertain the essential meaning(s) of a stated phenomenon (Creswell, 1998; Moustakas, 1994). The meaning must be derived from individuals who have lived the experience of the phenomenon. In an attempt to uncover the lived experience rehabilitation professionals were identified as having had first hand experience of religion and spirituality. There was no expectation about the quality of the experience nor was it relevant whether the experience was positive or negative. According to Polkinghorne (1988) the "narrative is the primary way through which humans organize their experiences into temporally meaningful episodes" (p. 1). In Spring 2001 fifteen rehabilitation professionals participated in answering semi-structured questions during audiotaped, in-depth interviews lasting 90 to 120 minutes each. The interviews took place in five US cities in three states. The study proposed three primary questions: (1) how do you define spirituality; (2) how do you define religion; and (3) how do you use these concepts in practice? This article focuses on the results of the third question.

Sampling

This study utilized purposeful sampling (Glaser & Strauss, 1967) and had two sampling goals. The first was locating participants who offered not only an interest in the topic but also were believed to have a wide scope and range of information about spirituality and religion. The second goal was to ensure that information-rich respondents were available to generate the information upon which the emergent design could be based (Guba & Lincoln, 1985). This purposeful strategy allowed for the development of a rich, thick view of the complexities associated with spirituality and religion. An effort was made to locate individuals interested in spirituality and/or religion as it related to rehabilitation practice, but not necessarily only those who thought the concepts should be utilized. Respondents were added until there was redundancy.

Respondents were individuals whom agreed to engage in first-person conversations (interviews) about the meaning of spirituality and/or religion and in what ways do they believe they use these strategies in practice. Table 1 highlights participant characteristics.

TABLE 1. Demographics of Respondents

Respondent	Gender	Ethnicity	Current Religion	Education	Experience (Yrs.)
P 1	M	C	Jewish	MSW/PHD	21
P 2	F	C	Christian	MA/Rehab.	7.5
P 3	M	African American	Baptist	MSW	9
P 4	F	C	Episcopalian	MA Counseling/ PHD/ABD	16
P 5	M	C	Non Denominational	MA/Sp. Ed.	35
P 6	M	C	Agnostic	MSW	39
P 7	M	C	Agnostic	PHD/Psych.	25
P 8	F	C	Christian	MA/Rehab.	3
P 9	F	E. Indian	Catholic	BS OT	19
P 10	F	C	Non Denominational	AA/Message Therapy	10
P 11	M	C	Catholic	MSW	30
P 12	F	C	Christian	MA/Rehab.	32
P 13	M	C	Christian	BA Business/ Sub Abuse	7
P 14	F	C	Catholic	MA/Sp. Ed.	23
P 15	M	Hispanic	Atheist	AA/PT	6

Data Collection

Data collection and analysis progressed in three general stages of data collection; the initial interview, the review of the interview transcripts (by respondents), and the review of the interpretations. At all three stages respondents were encouraged to make changes, suggestions, and corrections. Interviews were completed using a semi-structured interview protocol that was modified as data emerged with each sequential interview and occurred in the private homes of the respondents, the respondent's workplace, a conference center, and the interviewer's office. There was on-going interaction between the researcher, participants. During the interview respondents discussed their thinking about the use of these concepts and identified the strategies they utilized in their practice. The first themes began to emerge after the first interview and continued to blossom during the process.

Analysis

Analysis began when the first contact was made with a respondent and remained fluid throughout the process. In order to ensure the accuracy of the dialogues, summaries were written immediately after each session. Next, a review of the audiotape was completed and notes were extended and corrected. Each tape was reviewed a minimum of four times during the analysis. These tapes provided referent materials to check and compare with the researcher's memory, notes, and reflections. A professional transcriber was utilized. Tapes were reviewed while reading along with the transcripts. Memos and diagrams were used to conceptualize the data (Strauss & Corbin, 1998). Each document and interview protocol sported a header with date, demographics, and a code name given to each participant. Notes were utilized to produce conceptual labels, paradigm features, and indications of process that are discussed in results. Conditional matrixes were developed to understand the emerging dimensions, relationships, and variations of the emerging themes. These strategies and techniques helped to maintain focus. This process was repeated for all initial interviews. After all interviews were finalized and preliminary themes developed, the preliminary themes were returned to each participant so they could review the resulting themes as they emerged. The second level of analysis continued with the development of themes as new interviews were completed. The participants were invited to continue to comment as the process evolved, helping to co-create the essential meaning of spirituality and religion.

Trustworthiness was enhanced by regular reflection between the participants and the researcher as the data emerged (called member checks). The participants were offered the opportunity to reviewed their final individual narratives reflecting their stories. According to Guba and Lincoln (1985), member checks are "the most crucial technique for establishing credibility" (p. 314). Some respondents did not provide feedback. Technical writing and word choice concerns were modified to agree with the respondent's request. Another strategy utilized to minimize potential presuppositions during analysis was the use of external peer debriefings (Guba & Lincoln, 1985). Three peers (a colleague, a disinterested friend, and a colleague who had experience with phenomenology) reviewed all transcripts, the emerging analysis, and the resulting narratives. Each provided feedback suggesting alternative meanings to be considered.

FINDINGS

How Do You Use Spirituality or Religion in Practice?

First, respondents were asked to identify what they believed spiritual and or religious strategies in rehabilitation would be. Secondly, participants were asked if they used any spiritual or religious strategies in their rehabilitation practices. Initially most participants did not think they utilized any spiritual or religious strategies in rehabilitation practice. The interviews progressed in such a manner that their discovery usually followed a general pattern. First there was the initial discussion where they shared that they did not use the concepts in practice. Next was the consideration that they did use the strategies, but as a tool for benefitting themselves, to help them conceptualize their work with a particular client. With this awareness came the realization that they also practiced these activities directly with clients for the benefit of the client. I have presented the emergent themes in the order in which they evolved during the interviews.

Theme 1: Denial of Applying Spiritual or Religious Strategies

Initially, with the exception of P4, all participants denied engaging in any spiritual or religious activities with their clients. P4 did not hesitate to say she used the concepts in practice. When a client brought up the subject in some direct way each respondents made a very brief and limited intervention such as listening to the client before the professional tactfully changed the subject.

Most respondents reported ambivalent and conflicted ideas and feelings toward using these concepts in practice. Even when P8 believed it would be beneficial to a client she said, "I don't ever bring up religion with any person that I'm working with . . . I am not going to discuss with them religious or spiritual issues." As a state employee, she said there is a "constant tug of war inside me." If they did bring it up "I would try to steer the conversation away." When follow-up questions were posed she said that if she were in a religious setting that "would be totally different because then that would be an appropriate place to do that." Another typical response was given by P11 who stated simply "I don't really get into religion . . . unless it is demographic [*such as a question asked on an intake form*]."

An expressed reason for not asking centered on confusion about separation of church and state. P12 said, "I take very seriously the separation of church and state so I very hard try not to influence people." To illustrate she said:

> There were a couple of support groups that started in my area that I helped start that wound up meeting in churches . . . so I made sure to talk with my supervisor about 'Is this all right?' . . . One group did a collection each week and then every now and then if we had too much money we'd give it to the church and if we had potluck we invited the minister and the secretary . . . I talked to my supervisor about it and he said, 'Don't worry about it' and I said, 'Okay, I'm covered and I've discussed it.'

P12 worked with individual with low vision and blindness. Another example highlighted her confusion for the separation. She said, "There is an organization that gives a recorded Bible out free to anybody who is legally blind, so I tell all my clients about it, but I am very careful to say you don't have to take it if you don't want it."

The fear of pushing their beliefs on others was another reason participants voiced not offering spiritual or religious interventions. P8 had an experience early on that reinforced this idea for her.

> I had a student one time who was Mormon or Jehovah Witness, I can't remember which one, but she didn't like my crucifix that I was wearing and she said that it was offensive to her . . . I just turned it around and put it on the back of my neck so she didn't have to see it.

She said, "I don't want them to feel like, if I don't believe the way she does then she's not going to give me services."

Theme 2: Self Benefits

The fears of openly using the concepts gave way to the realization that they did use spiritual and religious strategies to help themselves while working as rehabilitation professional. Seven respondents made comments about being unable to separate themselves from their religious or spiritual lives. For example, P8 related, "I just think that religion is so much a part of me I can't really tease that apart from when I'm doing my job . . . it's such a part of me it is impossible to separate." P11 said, "my life is a prayer, if you know what I mean . . . there is no other way [*for me*] to be with clients when you think about it." He went on to say that for him working with people with disabilities meant he had to first come to some existential understanding of the situation at hand. He said his "own personal belief system and his faith was directly related to his peace of mind and how he practiced with his clients." In fact, "my belief system is why I am in the helping profession . . . There's a lot of needless suffering in the world . . . I see myself in the world but not of it . . . whatever comes and goes comes and goes." Religion helped him to continue in this important and sometimes painful work.

In four respondents self-benefit was framed around the issue of burnout. P2 said it best, "My religious beliefs have always been something that whenever things get tough, I cling to." She described having a position working with serious persistently mentally ill patients. "They just didn't get better in that system." She began to feel frustrated and alone by the daily grind, lack of visible positive outcomes or support for her work. She questioned herself. She found herself wondering how she fit into the universe and what was her purpose. She said,

> My Christian faith is what got me through. I believed Jesus had a difficult time and that he went through some things that were unjustified and that he managed to survive and grow stronger through all the adversity that he faced, which helped me know I could make it through. I was not alone.

P5 raised to the issue of spiritual and religious beliefs being an inoculation for burnout using Mother Theresa as an example saying, "Mother Theresa is filled with the primacy that she is there to serve and to share the love of the spirit–that these people are primary and everything else is secondary." It is ability to get a perspective of what is really is important which frees one up from secular expectations and allows the job to be more rewarding. "Mother Teresa was not burned out."

Two of the six respondents with their own disabilities said that their spiritual and religious practices helped them in their own adjustment to disabilities. Right before her accident P10 woke up in the hospital and called out God's name. "I saw him holding me. I was in so much pain and I should have died but my prayers and my underlying belief in God's healing powers saved my life." P8 also used her spiritual and religious beliefs to adjust to her significant learning disabilities saying:

> Now I know why I would sit in class in grade school if I were in the back I didn't pay attention. I had a learning disability . . . It made a lot of things fall into place and for me it made it okay to accept it

because I felt like God had a plan for my life; and if this is part of my life that was okay and I was able to put it in perspective.

Theme 3: Client Benefits

As the interview process progressed, thirteen participants had begun talking about the benefits of using spiritual or religious strategies in the rehabilitation process. These respondents believed that the outcome for adjustment to disabilities would be enhanced significantly if such strategies were employed. An interesting feature about the manner in which these respondents described the benefits to clients was related to good trust building and therapeutic techniques taught during educational and training programs. The surprise was not so much that they used them but that they described them as spiritual or religious. P2 made several comments regarding how spirituality or religion can positively affect a person's coping or adjustment.

> It's surprising to me the attitude of some of the people who have the more severe physical disabilities, that they have obviously found their own spirituality . . . they are more uplifted . . . [*if*] they have the background in spirituality or religion, that becomes a sense of comfort for them. . . . They tend to be more positive; they're looking at 'What can I do?' [*or*] 'I'm willing to do anything' kind of attitude.

P5 added that if "you have someone . . . who does have a strong spiritual foundation [*they are*] just so much better off than people who don't." When asked how engaging in faith, belief, religion, or spiritual discussions or interventions might affect adjustment for a client P8 said, "I'm sure they can [*adjust*] . . . just not very well."

According to the respondents, the very nature of a helping relationship calls for person-to-person contact. It usually involves some crisis or problem for which the client seeks assistance. This relationship is expected to be different from other social encounters with the benefits of the relationship being focused on the client. It requires special considerations including, but not limited to, a requirement for ethical and moral behaviors on the part of the helper. For six respondents, this moral and ethical approach gets its authority from some religious tradition or teachings and is, by its very practice, spiritual. In fact, the concept of helping or serving was associated with religious teachings and traditions of Judaism, Christianity, and Buddhism. Each participant came to an awareness of this and reported a number of examples of the ethical and moral client worker interaction.

Looking at the client as a whole human being was frequently used as an example of this. It was considered important for the respondents to look at the client as more than a 'disability,' 'illness,' or 'condition.' It was reasoned that to consider the whole person meant that the professional had to consider a bigger or broader view of how to assist the client. P5 related this in the following story,

> If we spent more time getting people as integrated and whole as possible, helping them as whole human beings, then they're going to be better able to handle . . . life's challenge. . . . I had a client with cystic fibrosis and she had just gotten out of the hospital . . . they called her a case number as opposed to [*name*]. . . . She said to me 'I really get tired of that because I'm a human being.' I knew this but it was reinforced by her and so many others . . . sometimes I had to stop and think, what is this person's disability?

P2 expressed it this way. "Rehabilitation means not just looking at one thing but rather the whole person and spirituality is part of that." This was also related to the idea of being more than a bean counter or bureaucrat. In spite of the "pressure we get from our higher ups" to be task oriented and to close cases, "I try . . . from the very beginning to let people know that I'm willing to do whatever I can to help them throughout their training program whether it has to do with school, like tutoring, or whether it has to do with just family pressures," related P2. P2 agreed with others that focusing on the whole person, instead of just a disability or task, was not only professionally and personally more rewarding, it also helped the individual client to achieve a better rehabilitation outcome.

According to the participants the right to self-determination and "starting where the client is" was seen as essential to making a connection and benefitting the client. By following these principles participants believed they could build a foundation of trust that would also benefit the client. For P3, leaves his "sterile" office environment to work on the streets to work with homeless vets stating, "I respect this other person's right to choose a different path and that it has to be about *caring* for the other person as opposed to imposing your will." He discovered that if he imposed his will to get them off the streets he was actually disrespecting the client's ability to make informed choices. This is "a disenfranchised population" and to work with them on their own terms means, "you cannot help but feel there's a spiritual connection." It is more of a "connection as a personal thing versus something that I'm doing as a job." Another example of this was shared by P6 who described that in his early years of practice he worked with a young boy diagnosed as schizoid and who had a very poor long-term prognosis.

> He was a very isolated little boy and would come into the clinic and sit next to my desk in a chair and if we said five words in the course of 45 minutes it would be absolutely a miracle. This went on eight to ten months. Years later I was in a grocery store and this fellow was checking groceries . . . and he recognized me and told me who he was, that he had gotten married, had a couple of kids and how incredibly helpful I had been . . . I said, 'You know, I don't really understand that at all' and he said the fact there was somebody just willing to sit and wait for me just made me feel so incredibly important . . . so he decided he was important.

Additionally five respondents introduced the idea that you must love your client. To see them as another human being, or as a child of God was a technique that helped the respondent engage with clients that were difficult to like, much less work with. P3 described it this way, "you have to love your patient. . . . You have to care for your patient. . . . But a lot of times it's not about that particular patient because they don't look very loveable . . . it's just really [*important to*] cherish humanity." P5 believed, "it's an internal perspective, it's a way to see people" and if the rehabilitation professional would treat clients with this attitude it would positively "affect the way they perceive you . . . the system and what happens to them." He did not believe it took extensive involvement and it was always reciprocal. He described an incident that happened to him to make his point that being there and showing love for someone you are helping can make a tremendous difference. He went to the library as a young boy and the librarian

> looked down at me and said, 'May I help you?' and there was love pouring from her eyes . . . she said four words and I felt bathed in love . . . it was a very big deal. That was 50 years ago and I can't think about it without my heart being touched [*he is crying telling this story*] . . . it's really more open to let the love shine through you . . . and if you give love to another person, if you give love to them then you've given them a gift and I also believe in the spiritual principle that in giving you receive. . . .

Closely related to the idea of loving, over half of the respondents used a "strengths perspective" to work with a client. This idea was presented in two ways. On the one hand, being spiritual or religious could be a very positive part of a person's life and by bringing these resources into the therapeutic relationship you could mobilize their helpful effects. P4 summarized her thinking about strengths by emphasizing what strengths the client comes with. If religion or spiritual beliefs or activities have worked for the client in the past "I work from that strength . . . [*I*] use that strength to successfully solve the problem that's in front of them right now." The other way to look at strengths of a spiritual or religious nature is to see it as a cultural and or diversity issue. P9 used three different cultural and religious groups to highlight this idea.

> India tends to be a lot more spiritual than here [*U.S.*] because it's very much a part of life . . . it's not something that's kept separate. . . . In Canada too, people talk about it more and it's not considered taboo . . . they are usually Catholic or Protestant. . . . The Hindus in India are a little more fatalistic about life . . . and as such, the people tend to be a little too fatalistic accepting the disability . . . but on the other hand, parents openly talk about praying to God. . . . I have a lot of Hispanic kids and I know they're a deeply religious people, usually Catholic, and with some of their mothers they have actually approached that and talked about it, and talked about faith . . . they seem more accepting of their children's disabilities . . . and they seem more open to talking about spirituality and religion than the other races that I [*currently*] work with.

Respondents also said they believed self-determination benefitted clients. It was seen as a spiritual way to connect. P10 said it this way:

> I have learned a lot through experience and I truly believe that you have to heal yourself, before you can help others heal themselves. I can only share my own experience, I can relate to pain. People look at me and say, 'Well, Honey you're young. You shouldn't be hurting.' When I tell them about my accident they go, 'Oh, you are no stranger to pain.' I have pain every single day . . . I tell them what has worked for me.

While self-disclosure was considered beneficial to clients, respondents also pointed out that the self-disclosure needed to be for the benefit of the client and not the respondent.

Developing trust via honesty was seen as very beneficial to clients and was explained by P8 as something that she considered a foundational issue in her religious view.

> Being honest with them. . . . Honesty to me comes from growing up in church and being taught that you should be honest. . . . I think those are parts of my religious upbringing . . . you know going an extra mile for them . . . what would Jesus do if he were in this situation?

For these respondents religion and or spirituality are the basis for framing their responses to the questions. It was their beliefs that underlined decisions about how clients can most benefit from their interaction with the professional helper. The strategies they overtly used are presented as the fourth theme.

Theme 4: Integrating Spiritual and Religious Strategies

The first strategy deliberately used was to role model what they learned to be important ways people should interact with others. This role modeling was based on the teachings, philosophy and activities highlighted in their respective religious or spiritual traditions. This can be most clearly seen by P3 who walked the streets serving homeless people.

> Jesus went to the people . . . he didn't wait until he got to the temple . . . It was closed on Friday nights and Saturday. It is beyond saying 'What would Jesus do?' It's a part of me. If you're in a very sanitized clinical setting, [*they*] come in and we talk, then that doesn't really take a whole lot. I usually dressed this well . . . [*my clients*] I mean the odors, the human odors are horrific . . . but to be willing to endure that goes beyond saying you're doing this for the paycheck. Jesus was a mentor for that. Jesus went to the people.

P14 told a story of a 16-year-old Catholic Puerto Rican woman who enrolled at the university. Her mother came with her to assist with the transition since [*name*] was also a quadriplegic needing assistance. Since her accident [*name*] had turned away from God and the Church. Her mother wanted her to return to church and to her faith. [*Name*] was so angry she was not ready to deal with God or her faith yet, but complied with her mother's request to locate a church. They came to the Office for Students with Disabilities and met this respondent.

The student asked, 'Where is there a Catholic Church?' I was torn between maybe I should do something and 'What are you doing here? Are you going to be Saul and say I don't hear anything, or are you going to be Paul and say, yes Lord, I'll go do what you want me to do.'

P14 took a middle road approach (told her where the churches were but did not discuss her struggles with her) at the time, but said today she would be more willing to talk, take and participate in the religious journey this young woman was seeking.

Several respondents told stories from various traditions. Sometimes they told stories from their own tradition but often utilized stories across different traditions. P3 gave this example from a client who said, "I've done a lot of bad in my life." P3 then asked him:

> 'Well, do you know who Paul is?' and he said, 'Well, no.' Paul was a man who went about persecuting Christians, people that were working for Jesus and working for other people; he was just like persecuting them and then all of a sudden he had this change in his life to where he turned around and he blossomed into a beautiful person, one that was one of the prolific writers of the New Testament . . . God used him as a tool and nobody held that against him . . . even the Christians that were being persecuted did not hold that against him, I mean they embraced him. God, who he really offended, did not hold it against him. . . .

This respondent also used the stories of the prodigal son and David who committed all kinds of atrocities. He used other stories from different paradigms. He believed it was useful to tell these stories because people related to them.

Seven respondents spoke of the teachings and activities of Jesus and Buddha who spent their lives serving and teaching others to serve. P5 said there were two life problems he saw that created for him two goals. One was personal spiritual growth and the other was "service to others . . . I really saw that I was a servant I was to serve them." He believed after studying various religions and philosophies that service to others was a universal truth. For him it was a motivating factor in choosing his life's work and how he saw approached every encounter with others whether it was a client or a colleague. Respondents for the most part thought the very fact that they were serving others was spiritual and often had its roots in a religious paradigm.

Referrals to church, religious leaders, or organizations were given as an intervention under two circumstances. The first occurred when the respondent felt the subject should remain off limits in practice or if the needed knowledge was beyond the scope of their own abilities. P6 spoke about the subject being off limits in practice and needing to be referred. He put it this way:

> It's unethical practice . . . I'm opposed to it . . . it would be up to the client to bring in and the problem I have in talking to some people who are adding spirituality, is that they've really got an axe to grind . . . they're making religion out of therapy and I think that's wrong.

One respondent (P7) who attended formal training to be a priest said:

> My partner here is an Army Chaplain, he's reserve but he's pretty active, he's three days a week here and two days at a Lutheran church . . . if somebody's issues are core issues, their central issues are more religious or spiritual in nature, I may either consult with him or refer someone to him to deal with it because I don't have a particular expertise in that area.

Eight used prayer or meditation as a spiritual or religious intervention strategy. Some who prayed did so outside the direct contact with the client. In the case of P8 even if a client asked for prayers she would promise to do so at their prayer time but not in the office or in the direct contact. P4 and P9 prayed directly with clients. P4 told of her experience when it was her turn to present a teaching case to students at a Christian Counseling Center, watching through a one-way mirror. She prepared the students for the case as she would any other case telling them that part of the mutually established goals the client wanted was to pray at the beginning and end of each session. The respondent prayed first and then prayed at the end of the session. This presentation was a live event of an actual session.

> It was like I had said you're going to engage in intercourse behind the mirror . . . it was a long pause . . . it was bizarre and I felt uncomfortable and the students were like, 'well, why are you doing this . . . You ought to refer this to a priest.' One of the people, the supervisor in charge was a priest, and so I tried to use the priest to kind of break the ice so it could be a kind of learning thing for all of

us . . . I asked the priest, 'Well, Father, you do this all the time, what do you say when you pray?' He said, 'I always just say, "let us pray," and everybody kneels.'

P9 went to see a patient as a referral in a rehabilitation hospital. She was an elderly woman who didn't really want occupational rehabilitation and said she was ready to die. On her own, P9 asked:

'Is there something you want to talk about? Do you believe in prayer?' She said, 'You can pray for me' and so I said some of the prayers that we say in the Catholic faith. The last thing she told me was, 'You've done more for me in the five days I've been in the hospital than anybody else since I came here.' The next morning when I came back she had died.

Thirteen participants identified touching and or holding as a spiritual or religious strategy. P6 who was adamantly opposed to using any spiritual or religious strategies in practice defined his holding and touching of clients as spiritual in nature. As a therapist for severely disturbed children he often found touching and or holding critical to his work. He described his intervention with a foster care child who was adopted by the foster family.

They took this little boy in at age six. They . . . really worked with this kid . . . and they continue to bring him in for treatment, he was hyperactive, had a seizure disorder, neurologically damaged, was horribly abused, molested, and mistreated in the foster care system. I saw him eight years . . . He would come into my office. . . me in a chair and we're playing a game together . . . essentially I've got my arms around him and I'm holding him through this activity. It was the only way that was tolerable for him to ever get held, was to have this excuse.

P11 told this story:

I remember seeing an ICU nurse, at the very last moments of a patient, an older man nobody was there, one of these people who dies alone, she was holding his hand by herself while he's taking his last breaths, and I thought, 'Oh my God, this is too moving.' I mean to see these things that people don't know about.

Touching was also utilized by P8 who said she would in no way engage in any spiritual or religious act in her work environment. She told the story of how a student was having a heart attack in her office a year earlier.

> We called 911 and the police came out and the paramedics came out, but while we were waiting for all of that response, I just sat with her and said, 'Okay let's just breathe real quietly and let's kind of slow down a little bit.' I mean she was really panicking because it was very frightful to her . . . I just could not just let her lay here on the floor until somebody showed up so I just talked to her and . . . let's just go to a quiet place in your head . . . I touched her hand to help her. . . .

P11 forgot the story until he relayed it during the interview. It occurred in a hospital neonate intensive care unit (NICU). A very premature infant was going to die but was sustained on a respirator. The parents decided to remove the respirator. The female, African American pediatrician approached the staff and said to P11:

> We're going to talk to them about removing the respirator and I would like to have you there and I'll be there, and the nurse will be there and the parents and anybody else they would want . . . they were going to have a ceremony and I thought well 'what are we going to have?' We're going to have a goodbye prayer for this family because they'd mentioned to the doctor about their religion . . . they weren't officially religious but they were spiritual. They didn't have [*clergy*] and so this is what we did . . . I didn't initiate it, the physician initiated [*it*] . . . The parents held the baby while the technician removed the respirator from the baby and of course immediately the baby ceased breathing, and was deceased at which point the mother, father, myself, the doctor and the nurse all of whom were crying including the speaker, just weeping silently, then went out of the NICU over to a lounge area that was quiet . . . not only did the doctor initiate a prayer but the doctor baptized the baby with the parents' permission because it was important symbolically to the parents, and it still gives me chills when I talk about it because it was extremely moving for this family to go through this and necessary to help with the grieving and help whatever had to be helped . . . it had tremendous meaning to this

family and sad . . . and even as we talk about it [*now*] I know it is so sad, but beautifully sad. [*It was*] one of the beautiful moments in [*my*] career . . .

The last of the specific strategies that emerged had to do with aesthetics such as poetry, music, art, nature, exercise, and yoga. It also included solitude (vs. isolation). These were highlighted at least twice in every interview. All had used these different strategies as an adjunct to their rehabilitation work. By the end of the interview all included these as religious or spiritual strategies. While it was not entirely clear why respondents came to realize they utilized the concepts in practice with clients, the discussion during the interviews seemed to provide an opportunity for the respondents to reflect on their everyday interaction with clients and colleagues. This reflection seemed to promote insight and trust in the interview process on the part of the respondents.

DISCUSSION

Participants were asked if they used religious or spiritual strategies and to identify and describe what a spiritual or religious intervention would be if they were used in practice. Four themes surfaced. They included: (1) strategies are not used in practice; (2) used for self-benefit; (3) used for client benefit; and (4) integrating spiritual and religious strategies. Although the rehabilitation literature has called for the introduction of spiritual and religious concepts into practice, only two participants were aware of this. One participant was aware because her discipline (OT) in Canada had called for the national organization to make it part of its code of ethics. The other participant was aware that the American Psychological Association (APA) had a new division established for dialogue and research into the subject. None of the participants were aware of the empirical studies showing a positive relationship between healing and spirituality, religion, or belief (Benson, 1993, 1996; Matthews, Larson, & Barry, 1993). Three named *Anatomy of an Illness* (Cousin, 1991) as their only exposure to these ideas.

Initially, twelve respondents made comments about this interview being the first time they had ever formally thought about spirituality and or religion as it applied to their work. In fact, only respondents exposed to formal religious training thought about how religion might be involved in their work. Ten reported they appreciated the opportunity to have the discussion provided by this interview. While they could and did articulate personal times of having their own faith tested at work, they felt that if the subject were discussed at work, it would be tested more due to ensuing disagreements. In observing participants it became clear they were coming to new awareness of what role religion or spirituality plays in their everyday lives and how much it already influenced personal and work behavior. Thirteen were surprised how often the opportunity presented itself to use religion and spirituality in their helping role with clients.

Better Client Outcomes

Seven voiced belief religion or spirituality was an essential element in obtaining maximum benefit from the rehabilitation process a belief held across many disciplines (Benson & Spilka, 1973; Harvard Medical School, 1998; Joyce & Welldon, 1965; Marini, 1995) and yet the implication was they actually withheld something that could potentially benefit a client. They thought it would be pushing their values on the client, was against agency policy and or a violation of the establishment clause. Upon reflection the contradictions between what they believed would be helpful and what they would offer a client appeared to surprise most respondents. As this contradiction surfaced, respondents began to think deeper about these questions and their own actions in practice.

Taboo Subjects in the Helping Process

Another image painted by five respondents is to how they understood the inappropriateness of religion or spirituality in practice. They likened it to other taboo subjects politics and sex. These taboos were seen of as personal and private. At first glance this might seem odd. Policy, for example, has a long history of importance for individuals with disabilities. The need for self-advocacy or empowerment in the political arena has been well defined by Vash (1994, 1995), Lane (1992, 1995), and others. Sex, too, is considered a relevant and important issue to discuss with clients with disability or illness (Tepper, 2000). While both of these areas may require the rehabilitation professional to have specific knowledge they are important factors in rehabilitation and deserve attention. Perhaps the issue has more to do with lack of training, which might lead the professional to feel uncomfortable about approaching these topics with their clients. In many ways this is similar to the reaction people have to addressing suicidal issues. Usually the untrained person is afraid of asking the question directly for fear that the person will then commit suicide due to the mere suggestion. Once trained, the helper will know that the question is critical and that they are not imposing their will. The client does not kill himself or herself because the worker asks the question. While some clients may be offended by the question most are not. Those that are can understand that this is an important issue in the helping relationship. It is likely the same can be said for religion and spirituality.

The Right to Self-Determination

Additionally, there was a sense that by introducing religion or spirituality into the helping relationship it would diminish the individual's freedom of choice and right to self-determination. When encouraged to clarify this, nine came up with abortion, genetic engineering (including stem cell research), homosexuality, and euthanasia as hot button topics. To participants' way of thinking, religion forced values upon individuals, which would again weaken the client's right to self-determination. When asked in a follow-up question about whether they believed that could actually change someone's view on religion, they responded that it might influence the client. They gave the examples that included the client being offended, whereby the client may have felt as though they had to change in order to get the help they were seeking. While it is not easy to change attitudes, beliefs or values all but one respondent implied this was a real threat if spirituality or religion were a part of the helping process. Only one participant verbalized an awareness that religion wasn't the only way people established their attitudes or beliefs and therefore persons who were religious or atheist could equally oppose or support any issue including those that were identified by the respondents. Nor was there a stated concern for those clients who wished to use their religious belief in the helping process. Only one respondent voiced insight that if spirituality and religion were ignored when the client requested it they too were not being afforded their right to self-determination.

Lack of Training and Professional Guidelines

Arguably professional groups should retain the right to self-determine and decide the area(s) of practice their professionals will engage in and how these activities will be regulated and or sanctioned.

Not a single participant received even basic information regarding the issues of spirituality and or religion in rehabilitation practice during formal rehabilitation training and or education. While 14 of the participants remembered that the topic had crossed their minds; none of them had thoroughly considered these topics and how they might be relevant to rehabilitation practice. While many wanted to discuss the topic during their training it was rare for it to come up. Several, with hindsight, voiced a wish they had pursued their questions in the classroom setting yet even those that did bring it up during classroom discussion felt it was a 'taboo' subject. The active suppression or ignoring religion or spirituality seemed to be reinforced by the silence in the classroom by faculty. Six respondents remembered an isolated comment or incident in the classroom about these issues but in each case the discussion was accompanied by comments from instructors who voiced concerns about the risk of discussing these issues in the classroom. According to three respondents instructors went so far as to say that if anyone had asked about the comments they had made in class, they would deny the discussion ever occurred. Because clients presented problems associated with spiritual or religious concerns the respondents believed they were inadequately prepared to make helpful and appropriate interventions and even referral.

Silent Interventions and Isolation

These situations were isolating and often left the respondents with cognitive dissonance between the need, their formal knowledge, and the behavior they ultimately engaged in with the client. This discomfort often left them isolated. Rarely was there any discussion among colleagues about these events. At times they witnessed others engaging in spiritual or religious ways with their clients or they were a part of a group of professionals who dealt with a spiritual or religious issue. When they did not act or follow their instincts they looked back at the situation with regret. Yet, even under these circumstances they usually did not speak to each other about it or if they did, it was minimal.

The participants gave more in-depth descriptions of the strategies they used in practice. Many of these strategies are used to develop connection with others and self. These strategies have also been highlighted in the literature (Bergin & Pain, 1991; Matthews, Larson, & Barry, 1993). Individuals with disabilities have also said that spiritual and religious activities have helped them to cope, adjust, and to recover to the highest level possible (Bennett, 1995; Benson, 1996; Collipp, 1969; Matthews 1998). Respondents did engage in these interventions because they believed the client would have a better rehabilitation outcome even when at first they did not call it religious or spiritual.

Confusion, Mixed Messages, and Ambivalence

Another finding was the ambivalence and mixed messages respondents gave about using the strategies. The question was raised about whether rehabilitation professionals should ask a client if they can engage in spiritual or religious practices or whether these practices must be kept private and or done without the explicit permission of the client. On one hand, the participants believed you should always ask before doing something spiritual or religious (i.e., prayer) but on the other hand some had artwork by artists who presented religious themes (i.e., Chegall) in their offices. The ambivalence also arose for interventions like touching, hand holding, or holding and whether or not the professionals asked permission of the client first. Yet when a client or patient was unconscious some of the same respondents thought touching was permissible since the client was unaware. Even within the same participant the message was mixed and often contradictory. For example, one woman voiced her opinion that she would not have religious or spiritual artifacts in her office. Yet she had them in her office when her clients had low or no vision and could not see them. That her co-workers might see them presented her with no concern. Yet this particular respondent also voiced concern about doing the research interview in her government office.

Helping Is Spiritual

Eleven participants believed that the helping relationship itself was a spiritual relationship, and it was the relationship that was the catalyst for enduring change. Two participants specifically cited Carl Jung's (1933, 1938) idea that all problems are spiritual problems. Thus they reasoned, how could the true helping relationship not be spiritual? They spoke of the need to 'love' their clients, which is seen as genuine caring and concern. When they spoke further about this issue the participants arrived at a position in opposition to managed care system of service delivery. They saw this as "bean counting" and not a helpful or meaningful way to provide services in a large bureaucracy. They expressed the idea, that as managed care has been instituted, the personal nature of the relationship in the helping situation was significantly diminished. The focus was seen to be on cost containment, statistics, reports, and closures.

Seven strongly believed this method of approaching clients led to a revolving door of disgruntled and dissatisfied customers. In fact, they echoed the comments of Nicholls (1995), who called for the 'aesthetic renaissance' (p. 148) as a way to rehumanize the service delivery system. While a service or a task was completed and they quickly closed 'the case,' the underlying relationship was never formed. In their mind this left both the worker and the client dissatisfied. The client would return to get another need met that was missed or ignored in the previous go-around. Participants themselves have contemplated leaving the field to find something that was more fulfilling. This dialogue reflected the attitudes of those in the early 20th Century when discussing the values (including the idea of loving those served) espoused under the Social Gospel movement (Krueger, 1999).

New Insight for Participants

Overall it can be said that the participants went through three stages during the interview. In sequence all but one person went through the same process. The first step in the sequence was the initial denial of any and all use of spiritual or religious strategies. Second was awareness that they could not separate themselves from their spiritual or religious beliefs. Therefore, they did engage in spiritual or religious ways of behaving that enhanced their skills as rehabilitation professionals and were used in their own personal coping with this sometimes-difficult work (van der Kolk, McFarland, & Weisaeth, 1996). Third was the insight that they directly used the strategies in practice with clients. Related to this was the dawning belief that there should be more training while they were in school and on-going professional education once they left school. All considered that spirituality and religion were appropriate topics if for no other reason, it was a part of engaging in a culturally sensitive practice in a pluralistic society with differing religious practices and beliefs (Abramowitz, 1993; Al-Krenawi & Graham, 1996).

Future Research

Many questions arose during the study. Those that emerged during the interview were outside the scope of this study and should be explored in future research endeavors and have been outlined below. Those that resulted from the analysis highlighted the fact that there is much to learn about these issues related to rehabilitation practice. Since this research was exploratory it will be necessary to continue to develop our professional knowledge in this area. The gaps in our current understanding calls for a step-by-step progression of knowledge building in order to develop a solid understanding of the concepts and their usefulness in rehabilitation practice. Furthermore, it would helpful to understand how demographics such as age, gender, race, personal religious or spiritual orientation, and the type of professional training received (rehabilitation, special education, social work, psychology, occupational training, etc.) affect the responses individuals might have regarding the use of spirituality and or religion in rehabilitation practice. Additionally, the type of setting where the professional is employed (hospice, rehabilitation hospital, oncology, substance abuse, inpatient or outpatient, and public or private facilities, etc.) may make a significant difference in attitudes and use of the spiritual or religious strategies in practice.

It became clear that respondents lacked adequate awareness of religion and spirituality as they related to practice. Studies that assess current knowledge and comfort level with using the knowledge would help identify important teaching or training issues. Along with this, it may be useful to know if rehabilitation professionals are already applying these concepts in practice and what do they currently label them as?

Another question highlighted in the study is to what degree (if any) can talking about or introducing the concepts in practice changes the person influence the client's beliefs? To what degree do our clients see these issues as helpful, useless, or offensive? Does the introduction of these concepts in the helping relationship appear or feel coercive to the client? Would like clients like spirituality and or religion included in their rehabilitation experience? Under what circumstances and to what degree would they like the concepts applied? Under what circumstances should these concepts not be used in practice?

It seemed plausible that the strategies used by these respondents might be unique to these individuals. Would a larger random sample of rehabilitation professionals select the same strategies as spiritual or religious interventions? Would they engage in such activity with their clients present, not present, or not at all? If they did engage in them, under what conditions would this occur? Does the type of disability or the type of help sought make a difference in what strategies may be necessary?

Suggestions for Training and Education

Most respondents indicated a desire for more training and understanding of the concepts. Each respondent identified spiritual and religious issues and situations in their actual practices, which they did not feel they were adequately trained to address or handle. All suggested more classroom discussion about the topics. Additionally, since professionals are calling for the inclusion of these issues in practice and professionals are already using them to some degree, it seems relevant and appropriate for the profession itself to articulate, sanctify, standardize, and regulate what is appropriate in the field.

Minimally it is recommend that spirituality and religion should be infused in existing rehabilitation, health, or mental health course content or in a separate course (Larson, Lu, & Swyers, 1996). Course work might include the history of religion and spirituality (Conrad, 1980) in the helping professions. It should include both the positive and negative aspects of the relationship of religion and or spirituality to rehabilitation over time allowing an open, nonjudgmental discussion of the issues associated with these topics. This material should also include information on public policy especially around the issues of the establishment clause or separation of church and state with dialogue about the new focus on faith-based service intervention and delivery.

There should also be material presented about what the concepts mean, including those important common denominators across all religions. Students should be aware of the functions of religion and spirituality and the myths (Campbell, 1988) associated with these concepts through time. Students should be educated about the impact spirituality and religion has on health, wellness, healing (Benson, 1996; Campbell, 1988), adjustment (Burke, 1999; Guy, 1982; Levers & Maki, 1995), work (Spitznagel, 1992, 1997) and disability (Byrd, 1993, 1999; Havranek, 1995, 1998; Lane, 1992; Vash, 1995). When teaching other developmental theories it should also include the faith development theories such as Fowler (1981) as well. Informed and guided dialogues in the classroom about religion as a diversity issue should be addressed.

Since the rehabilitation field has moved toward a strength based perspective (vs. a deficient medically based model) it is critical to teach future professionals how these concepts may make contributions to the well being of the client and as well as the rehabilitation professional (Canda, 1998, 1999; Delgado & Humm-Delgado, 1982). With the ecological model of intervention as a main stay of practice, it is critical to teach students how to consider the whole person in their environment including religious and spiritual aspects of the individual. As the student becomes more aware of how these issues come together, it is then important to educate the student on the skills and specific techniques that may be used in relationship to spirituality and religion. Education about community resources and referral should be included as a part of the skill and technique portion of the training.

CONCLUSION

This study explored how fifteen rehabilitation professionals with at least three years of experience in rehabilitation used these concepts in practice. Four themes emerged: (1) denial of having used strategies; (2) respondents used the concepts for their own benefit; (3) respondents used the concepts for the benefit of the clients; and (4) they used a multitude of strategies with and without the client's presence or permission. Respondents also were surprised by their own use of the concepts in practice. While initially denying the use of these concepts in rehabilitation practice, 14 of the respondents came to the insight that they did utilize the concepts with their clients. While the circumstances varied, all used the spiritual and religious concepts in practice to benefit themselves, their work, and their clients. Respondents called for the inclusion of these concepts into their rehabilitation training. Finally, suggestions for future research have been made as well as a call to the profession to include formal education and training of these issues in the safe classroom environment.

REFERENCES

Abramowitz, L. (1993). Prayer as therapy among the frail Jewish elderly. *Journal of Gerontological Social Work*, 19(3/4), 69-75.

Al-Krenawi, A., & Graham, R. (1996). Social work and traditional healing rituals among the Bedouin of Negev, Israel. *International Social Work*, 39(2), 177-188.

Anderson, J., Anderson, L., & Felsenthal, G. (1993). Pastoral needs and support within an inpatient rehabilitation unit. *Archives of Physical Medicine and Rehabilitation*, 74 (6), 574-578.

Atkins, B. (1988). An asset-oriented approach to cross cultural issues: Blacks in rehabilitation. *Journal of Applied Rehabilitation Counseling*, 19(4), 45-49.

Axinn, J., & Levin, H. (1997). *Social welfare: A history of the American response to need. (4 Ed.)* NY: Longman.

Barbour, I. (1997). *Religion and science: Historical and contemporary issues.* NY: Harper-Collins.

Becvar, D. (1997). *Soul healing: A spiritual orientation in counseling and therapy.* NY: Basic Books.

Bennett, J. (1995). Prayer for healing in a state mental hospital. *Journal of Religion in Disability & Rehabilitation,* 2(1), 21-25.

Benson, H. (1993). Relaxation and other alternative therapies. *Patient Care,* 27, 75-86.

Benson, H. (1996). *Timeless healing: The power and biology of belief.* NY: Simon & Schuster.

Benson, P., & Spilka, B. (1973). God image as a function of self-esteem and locus of control. *Journal for the Scientific Study of Religion,* 12, 297-310.

Bergin, A,. & Pain, I. (1991). Proposed agenda for a spiritual strategy in personality and psychotherapy. *Journal of Psychology and Christianity,* 10(3), 197-210.

Brabeck, M. (Ed.). (1989). *Who Cares? Theory, research and educational implications of the ethic of care.* London: Praeger.

Burgener, S. (1994) Caregiver religiosity and well-being in dealing with Alzheimer's dementia. *Journal of Religion and Health,* 33(2), 174-189.

Burke, K. (1999). *Health, mental health, and spirituality in chronically ill elders.* IL: University of Chicago Press.

Burkett, S. (1977) Religion, parental influence, and adolescent alcohol and marijuana use. *Journal of Drug Issues,* 7(3), 263-273.

Byrd, K., & Byrd, P. (1993). A listing of biblical references to healing that may be useful as bibliotherapy to the empowerment of rehabilitation clients. *Journal of Rehabilitation,* 59(3), 46-50.

Byrd, K. (1999). Spiritual care matters: Application of helping theories and faith in the lives of persons with disabilities. *Journal of Religion, Disability, and Health,* 3(1), 3-13.

Cadwallander, H. (Ed.). (1991). Depression and religion. *Counseling and Values,* 35(2), entire issue.

Campbell, J. (1972). *Hero with a thousand faces.* Princeton University Press.

Canda, E. (1995). Spirituality: A special issue. *Reflections: Narratives of Professional Helping,* 1(4), 1-81.

Canda, E. (1998). *Spirituality and social work: New directions.* Binghamton, NY: Haworth Pastoral Press.

Canda, E., & Furman, L. (1999). *Spiritual diversity in social work practice: The heart of helping.* NY: Free Press.

Collipp, P. (1969). The efficacy of prayer: A triple blind study. *Medical Times,* 97, 201-204.

Comstock, G., & Partridge, K. (1972). Church attendance and health. *Journal of Chronic Diseases,* 25(12), 665-672.

Conrad, A. (1989). Developing an ethics review process in a social service agency. *Social Thought,* 15, 102-115.

Conrad, A. (1980). Social ministry in early church: An integral component of the Christian Community. *Social Thought,* 6(2), 41-51.

Cornett, C. (1998). The soul of psychotherapy: Recapturing the spiritual dimension in the therapeutic encounter. NY: Free Press.

Cousin, N. (1991). *Anatomy of an illness*. NY: Doubleday.

Creswell, J. (1998). *Qualitative inquiry and research design: Choosing among five traditions*. CA: Sage Pub.

Delgado, M., & Humm-Delgado, D. (1982). Natural support systems: Source of strength in Hispanic communities. *Social Work, 27*, 83-89.

Dudley, R., Mutch, P., & Cruise, R. (1987). Religious factors and drug usage among Seventh-Day Adventist youth in North America. *Journal for the Scientific Study of Religion, 26*(2), 218-233.

Dunajski, B. (1994). *Spirituality: The nurse's lived experience*. (Doctoral Dissertation, Adelphi University, 1994). University of Michigan Dissertation Services, AAT942 434 7.

Dunbar, H., Mueller, W., Medina, C., & Wolf, T. (1998). Psychological and spiritual growth in women living with HIV. *Social Work, 43*, 144-154.

Elie, M. (1995). Be still. *Rehabilitation Education, 9*(2), 183.

Fowler, J. (1981). *Stages of faith*. San Francisco, CA: Harper & Row.

Frankl, V. (1969). *Man's search for meaning*. NY: Simon & Schuster.

Frankl, V. (1986). *The doctor and the soul: From psychotherapy to logotherapy*. NY: Vintage Books.

Garske, G. (1999). The challenge of rehabilitation counselors: Working with people with psychiatric disabilities. *Journal of Rehabilitation, 65*(1), 21-26.

Ginsburg, M., Quirt, C., & Ginsburg, A. et al. (1995). Psychiatric illness and psychosocial concerns of patients with newly diagnosed lung cancer. *Canadian Medical Association Journal, 152*(5), 701-708.

Glasser, B., & Strauss, A. (1967). *Discovery of grounded theory: Strategies for qualitative research*. Chicago, IL: Aldine de Gruyter.

Goldberg, C. (1996). The privileged position of religion in the clinical dialogue. *Clinical Social Work Journal, 24*(2), 125-136.

Green, L., Fullilove, M., & Fullilove, R. (1998). Stories of spiritual awakening: The nature of spirituality in recovery. *Journal of Substance Abuse Treatment, 15*(4), 325-331.

Gregorie, K. (1995). Alcoholism: The quest for transcendence and meaning. *Clinical Social Work Journal, 23*(3), 339-359.

Guba, E., & Lincoln, Y. (1985). *Naturalistic inquiry*. Thousand Oaks, CA: Sage Publications.

Guy, R. (1982). Religion, physical disabilities, and life satisfaction in older age cohorts. *International Journal of Aging & Human Development, 15*(3), 225-232.

Haake, L. (1996). *Love made visible: A qualitative study of spiritually oriented clinical social work practice*. Unpublished master's thesis. Catholic University of America.

Harvard Medical School. (Ed.). (1998). *Spirituality and Healing in Medicine V*. Harvard Medical School, The Mind/Body Medical Institute Care Group, Beth Israel Deaconess Medical Center; Under the Direction of Herbert Benson, March 22-24, 1998; Houston, TX.

Havranek, J. (1995). The role of the Christian rehabilitation counselor in secular service settings. *Journal of Religion in Disability & Rehabilitation, 2*(3), 67-73.

Havranek, J. (1998). *The role of spirituality in the rehabilitation process: Impacts on clients and counselors.* Paper presented to the National Rehabilitation Association Annual Conference, Orlando, FL. December 5, 1998.

Havranek, J. (1999). The role of spirituality in the rehabilitation process: Impacts on clients and counselors. *Journal of Religion, Disability, & Health*, 3(2), pp. 15-35.

Holland, P. (1989). Values, faith, and professional practice. *Social Thought*, 15(1), 28-40.

Hunt, B. (1996). Rehabilitation counseling for people with HIV disease. *Journal of Rehabilitation*, 62(3), 68-75.

Idler, E., & Kasl, S. (1997a). Religion among disabled elderly persons I: Cross-sectional patterns in health practices, social activities, and well-being. *Journal of So-, cial Sciences.*

Idler, E., & Kasl, S. (1997b). Religion among disabled and non-disabled elderly persons II: Attendance at religious services as a predictor of the course of disability. *Journal of Gerontology: Social Sciences,* 52(6). pp. S-1294-S-1305.

Iorfido, B. (1996). Incorporating faith into the recovery model for a person with multiple personality disorder. *Social Work and Christianity*, 23(3), 87-101.

Jerotic, V. (1997). The role of religion in rehabilitation of psychiatric patients. *Psihijatrija Danas*, 29(3/4), 279-292.

Joyce, D., & Welldon, R. (1965). The efficacy of prayer: A double-blind clinical trial. *Journal of Chronic Disease*, 18, 367-377.

Jung, C. (1933). *Modern man in search of a soul.* NY: Harcourt, Brace, Jovanovich Publishers.

Jung, C. (1938). *Psychology and religion.* New Haven, CT: Yale University Press.

Kaczorowski, J. (1989). Spiritual well-being and anxiety in adults diagnosed with cancer. *Hospice Journal*, 5(3/4), 105-116.

Kaplan, M., Marks, G., & Mertens, B. (1997). Distress and coping among women with HIV infection: Preliminary findings from a multiethnic sample. *American Journal of Orthopsychiatry*, 67(1), 80-91.

Krill, D. (1990b). Reflections on teenage suicide and adult addictions. *Spirituality and Social Work Communicator*, 1(1), 10-11.

Kruger, A. (1999). A personal reflection: The Social Gospel and the Canadian *Social Work Code of Ethics. Canadian Social Work*, 1(1), 25-29.

Landis, B. (1996). Uncertainty, spiritual well-being, and psychosocial adjustment chronic illness. *Issues in Mental Health Nursing*, 17, 217-231.

Lane, N. (1992). A spirituality of being: Women with disabilities. *Journal of Applied Rehabilitation Counseling*, 23(4), 53-58.

Lane, N. (1995). A theology of anger when living with disability. *Rehabilitation Education*, 9(2), pp. 97-111.

Larson, D., Lu, F., & Swyers, J. (Eds.). (1996). *Model curriculum for psychiatric residency training programs: Religion and spirituality in clinical practice.* MD: National Institute for Healthcare Research.

Larson, D., & Larson S. (1994). *The forgotten factor in physical and mental health: What does the research show?* Rockville, MD: National Institute for Healthcare Research.

Levers, L., & Maki, D. (1995). African indigenous healing and cosmology: Toward a philosophy of ethnorehabilitation. *Rehabilitation Education*, 9(2), pp. 127-145.

Lindberg, C. (1993). *Beyond charities: Reformation initiatives for the poor.* Minneapolis, MN: Fortress Press

Marini, I. (1995). Spiritual and psychological correlates of adjusting to traumatic injury. *Journal of Religion in Disability & Rehabilitation*, 2(1), 67-71.

Matthews, D. (1998). *The faith factor: Proof of the healing power of prayer.* NY: Viking.

Matthews, D., Larson, D., & Barry, C. (1993). *The faith factor: An annotated bibliography of clinical research on spiritual subjects. Vol. 1.* Rockville, MD. National Institute for Healthcare Research.

Matthews, D., & Saunders, D. (1997). *The faith factor: An annotated bibliography of clinical research on spiritual subjects, Vol. IV: Prevention and treatment of illness, addictions, and delinquency.* Rockville, MD: National Institute for Healthcare Research.

McCarthy, H. (1995b). Understanding and reversing rehabilitation counseling's neglect of spirituality. *Rehabilitation Education*, 9(2), 187-199.

Miller, W. (1998). Researching the spiritual dimensions of alcohol and other drug problems. *Addiction*, 93(7), 979-990.

Morell, C. (1996). Radicalizing recovery: Addiction, spirituality and politics. *Social Work*, 41, 306-312.

Morrison-Orton, D. (In Press). How rehabilitation professionals define the concepts of spirituality and religion when working with individuals with disabilities. *Journal of Social Work in Disability & Rehabilitation*.

Moustakas, C. (1994). *Phenomenological research methods.* Thousand Oaks, CA: Sage.

Nicholls, R. (1995). Pragmatic spirituality: Enablement in traditional Africa. *Rehabilitation Education*, 9(2), pp. 147-158.

O'Brien, M. (1982). Religious faith and adjustment to long-term hemodialysis. *Journal of Religion, Disability, & Health*, 21(1), 68-80.

O'Hanlon, W. (1999). *Solution-oriented therapy for chronic and severe mental illness.* NY: John Wiley Publishing.

Olasky, M. (1992). *The tragedy of American compassion.* Washington, DC: Regnery Press.

Patton, M. (1990). (2nd ed.). *Qualitative evaluation and research methods.* Thousand Oaks, CA: Sage.

Paykel, E., Myers, J., Lindenthal, J., & Tanner, J. (1974). Suicidal feelings in the general population: A prevalence study. *British Journal of Psychiatry*, 124, 460-469.

Peck, S. (1993). *A world waiting to be born: Civility rediscovered.* NY: Bantam Books.

Pellebon, D., & Anderson, S. (1999). Understanding the life issues of spirituality-based clients. *Families in Society*, 80(3), 229-238.

Pezzulo, J. (1997). *Social workers' clinical decisions regarding religious and spiritual issues in direct practice: A quantitative analysis.* Unpublished doctoral dissertation. University of Pittsburgh.

Polkinghorne, D. (1988). *Narrative knowing and the human sciences.* Albany, NY: State University of New York.

Reid, N., & Popple, R. (Eds.). (1992). *The moral purposes of social work: The character and intentions of a profession.* Chicago: Nelson-Hall.

Rogers, C. (1942). *Counseling and psychotherapy.* Boston: Houghton Mifflin.

Rotteveel, J. (1999). When God Isn't Santa Claus. *Journal of Religion, Disability, & Health,* 3(1), 49-54.

Sheehan, W., & Kroll, J. (1990). Psychiatric patients' belief in general health factors and sin as causes of illness. *American Journal of Psychiatry,* 147, 112-113.

Sheridan, J. (1995). Honoring angels in my path: Spiritually-sensitive group work with persons who are incarcerated. *Reflections: Narrative of Professional Helping,* 1(4), 5-16.

Simons, B. (1992). Acknowledging spirituality in recovery: A mental health consumer's perspective. *Spirituality and Social Work Journal,* 3(1), 5-7.

Sistler, A., & Washington, K. (1999). Serenity for African American caregivers. *Social Work with Groups,* 22(1), 49-62.

Skocpol, T. (1995). *Protecting soldiers and mothers: The political origins of social policy in the United States.* MA: Harvard Press.

Smith, E. D., Stefanek, E., Joseph, V., & Verdieck, J. (1993). Spiritual awareness, personal perspective on death and psychosocial distress among cancer patients: An initial investigation. *Journal of Psychosocial Oncology,* 11(3), 89-103.

Spitznagel, R. (1992). The spiritual dimension in holistic adjustment services. *Vocational Evaluation and Work Adjustment Bulletin, Monograph,* 100-101.

Spitznagel, R. (1997). Spirituality in work adjustment: A dimension to be considered. *Vocational Evaluation and Work Adjustment Bulletin,* Winter, 111-117.

Stern, R., Canda, E., & Doershuk, F. (1992). Use of non-medical treatment by cystic fibrosis patients. *Journal of Adolescent Health,* 13, 612-614.

Strauss, A., & Corbin, J. (1998). *Basics of qualitative research: Techniques and procedures for developing grounded theory.* (2nd ed.). Thousand Oaks, CA: Sage Publications.

Sullivan, P. (1992). Spirituality as social support for individuals with severe mental illness. *Spirituality and Social Work Journal,* 3(1), 7-13.

Taylor, K., & Wolfer, T. (1999). Social work as a vocation: Balancing ministry and profession. *Social Work and Christianity,* 26(1), 112-126.

Tepper, M. (2000). Sexuality and disability: The missing discourse of pleasure. *Sexuality and Disability,* 18(4), 283-290.

Tratter, W. (1994). *From Poor Law to welfare state.* NY: Free Press.

Trieschmann, R. (1995). The energy model: A new approach to rehabilitation. *Rehabilitation Education,* 9(2), 217-227.

van der Kolk, B., McFarlane, A., & Weisaeth, L. (1996). *Traumatic stress: The effects of overwhelming experience on mind, body, and society.* NY: Guilford Press.

van Wormer, K. (1997). *Social Welfare: A worldview.* Chicago: Nelson-Hall.

Vash, C. (1981). *The psychology of disability.* NY: Springer Publishing Co.

Vash, C. (1994). *Personality and adversity: Psychospiritual aspects of rehabilitation.* NY: Springer.

Vash, C. (1995). Metaphysical influences on disability attitudes. *Rehabilitation Education,* 9(2), 113-127.

Walsh, J. (1995). The impact of schizophrenia on clients' religious beliefs: Implications for families. *Families in Society*, 76(9), 551-558.

Wuthnow, R., & Hodgkinson, A. (1990). *Faith and philanthropy in America: Exploring the role of religion in America's voluntary sector.* San Francisco: Jossey-Bass.

Yates, J., Chalmer, B., & St. James, P. et al. (1981). Religion in patients with advanced cancer. *Medical and Pediatric Oncology*, 9(2), 121-128.

Medication of Children and Youth in Foster Care

Diane L. Green
Wesley Hawkins
Michelle Hawkins

SUMMARY. This study examined the type and frequency of prescribed medication of foster care youth in a south Florida county during April, 2001. Using file reviews and structured interviews with targeted case managers, it was found that 23% of the total sample (n = 722) were currently using medication. Most frequent medications prescribed were Risperdal, Clonidine, Adderall, and Ritalin. The majority of subjects had multiple prescriptions (57%) with no one pattern found for multiple prescribed drugs. The most frequent behaviors and symptoms found for those prescribed medication were sadness, delinquency history, and argumentative behavior. Approximately three-fourths of the youth had medications monitored, while the most frequent schedule of monitoring

Diane L. Green, PhD, is Assistant Professor, Wesley Hawkins, PhD, is Professor, and Michelle Hawkins, PhD, is Professor and Director, Florida Atlantic University, School of Social Work, 777 Glades Road, P.O. Box 3091, Boca Raton, FL 33341.

Address correspondence to: Diane Green, PhD, 6016 Edgemere Court, Palm Beach Gardens, FL 33410 (E-mail: dgreen@fau.edu).

This study could not have been completed without the help of Pat Rowland who is the Assistant Director of Field at Florida Atlantic University and Mary Chi, a graduate student at Florida Atlantic University.

[Haworth co-indexing entry note]: "Medication of Children and Youth in Foster Care." Green, Diane L., Wesley Hawkins, and Michelle Hawkins. Co-published simultaneously in *Journal of Social Work in Disability & Rehabilitation* (The Haworth Social Work Practice Press, an imprint of The Haworth Press, Inc.) Vol. 4, No. 1/2, 2005, pp. 43-55; and: *Disability Issues for Social Workers and Human Services Professionals in the Twenty-First Century* (ed: John W. Murphy, and John T. Pardeck) The Haworth Social Work Practice Press, an imprint of The Haworth Press, Inc., 2005, pp. 43-55. Single or multiple copies of this article are available for a fee from The Haworth Document Delivery Service [1-800-HAWORTH, 9:00 a.m. - 5:00 p.m. (EST). E-mail address: docdelivery@haworthpress.com].

was monthly. The foster care placement was most likely to monitor medication while a psychiatrist did almost all prescribing. The most frequent placement was therapeutic foster home while the most frequent Diagnostic and Statistical Manual diagnoses were Attention Deficit Hyperactivity Disorder, Post Traumatic Stress Disorder, Major Depression, and Bi-Polar Disorder. One most striking finding for mental health was that those currently on medication were much more likely to have been Baker Acted (Florida law that provides a reasonable process for involuntarily committing those whose conduct makes them dangerous to themselves or others) than non-medication foster care youth. Finally, few barriers to services were found for the medication sample in receiving medication services. *[Article copies available for a fee from The Haworth Document Delivery Service: 1-800-HAWORTH. E-mail address: <docdelivery@ haworthpress.com> Website: <http://www.HaworthPress. com> © 2005 by The Haworth Press, Inc. All rights reserved.]*

KEYWORDS. Foster care, prescription drugs, mental health, depression, Baker Act, youth

PHARMACOTHERAPY WITH CHILDREN: BRIEF BACKGROUND

Combined pharmacotherapy, which includes the use of psychotropic medications with traditional therapeutic techniques, has become an important and innovative component in the therapeutic arena (Wilens, Biederman, Mick, & Spencer, 1995). Despite the positive trend for pharmacotherapy, there exists literature on adverse drug reactions in the use of psychotropics in children (Bhatara, Kallepalli, Misra, & Awadallah, 1996; Cantwell, Swanson, & Connor, 1997; Fenicel, 1995; Popper & Zimnitzky, 1995). Woolston (1999) found major pitfalls in using medication with or without combined therapeutic treatments:

(a) Physicians often rely on secondhand reports rather than direct examination of the patient, (b) medication regimens begin after one single visit, (c) follow-up monitoring is brief and infrequent, (d) monitoring treatment is done over the telephone, and (e) many physicians do not integrate pharmacotherapy with psycho-social approaches. (p. 1,456)

This practice places the identified patient or client with the blame. Environmental factors are not taken into consideration. As Woolston (1999) noted, this is unacceptable since children are more dependent than adults in terms of their flexibility with stressors.

PREVALENCE

An anonymous survey found that 95 percent of medical practitioners used pharmacotherapy for posttraumatic stress disorder as the major therapeutic modality (Cohena, Mannarinoa, & Rogalb, 2001). In 1997 children between the ages of 6 and 18 years received 792,000 prescriptions for selective serotonin reuptake inhibitors (SSRIs) alone (Hoar, 1998). Hoar (1998) also found during this same period, the number of children aged 5 and younger taking these medications jumped 500 percent, from 8,000 to 40,000. Another survey by the University of North Carolina at Chapel Hill School of Medicine (1999) found that 72 percent of family physicians and pediatricians acknowledged having prescribed an SSRI for patients under 18 years old. Of these, eight percent reported having adequate training, and 16 percent reported feeling comfortable treating depression in children. Eighty percent of all medication used in children is estimated to be "off-label" (Jensen, Bhatara, & Vitello, 1999).

Testing for the safety and efficacy of medications designed for adults, yet prescribed for children with similar diagnoses, has not been utilized. "Off-label" prescribing further demonstrates concerns for safety and efficacy in children. Studies by Geller, Reising, and Leonard (1999) and Storch (1998) reveal significant benefits to psychotropic medications used in children and adolescents for a variety of different diagnoses. However, these are limited in that they don't address the efficacy of commonly "off-labeled" prescriptions. Implementing studies for children is important, but not always feasible.

CAN FINDINGS FROM PHARMACOTHERAPY STUDIES WITH ADULTS BE APPLIED TO CHILDREN?

Because children are continuously developing and growing, the results of data collected from adults are not necessarily applicable to youth (Vitiello, Jensen, & Hoagwooda, 1999; Jensen et al., 1999). Direct participation by subjects in research is crucial in obtaining reliable and valid data. While studies that directly involve children have been minimal and have been on the rise in more recent years, data remains limited and in sharp contrast to the advances in the adult field (*Journal of the American Academy of Child and Adolescent Psychiatry*, 1999; Vitiello et al., 1999). Diller (2000) expressed the challenges in obtaining meaningful data because diagnoses are ambiguous, drug effects are nonspecific, and obtaining data from samples in the general community is extraordinarily difficult. Vitiello et al. (1999) and Walkup, Labellarte, and Riddle (1998) also discussed the ethical dilemmas in studies involving child and adolescent psychiatry. Potential benefits, minimal risk, informed consent, and selection bias are ethical dilemmas that limit the feasibility of research with this population. Children in foster care experience even more obstacles to receiving mental health services.

ARE FOSTER CHILDREN MORE VULNERABLE?

When children are removed from their homes and placed into foster care, another set of variables is exposed and needs to be addressed. Child Protective Services (CPS) exists to ensure safety and well being for children who are abused, neglected, and abandoned. CPS workers exist to monitor and provide the resources and avenues for children that their primary caregivers were unable to meet. There is evidence that mental health components are under-evaluated when compared with physical health, despite the fact that foster children are at significant risk for behavioral and psychological problems (Leslie et al., 2000). Leslie et al. (2000) further state that national estimates equal over 500,000 children in foster care. Many of these children are members of minority populations and share backgrounds of chronic poverty, familial disruptions, stresses, and social problems, including substance abuse. Potential barriers in receiving accurate evaluations for ethnic minority children may include biased assessment techniques, cultural and language barriers, lack of knowledge about available services, and lack of minority mental health providers. The author further cites between 35% and 85% of children entering foster care have significant mental health problems. In California and Washington, foster care children were significantly more likely to receive both outpatient and inpatient mental health services than non-foster children (Takayama, Bergman, & Connell, 1994).

In a 1999 study of foster children in Los Angeles, children diagnosed with attention deficit/hyperactivity disorder were more than twice as high as those children in the community (Zima, Bussing, & Crecelius, 1999). Zima et al. (1999) also found that 16 percent had taken psychotropic medications sometime in their life. The results of this study could not be generalized to the greater population because of the socioeconomic variables of this major metropolitan area. Another limitation of the study was the absence of data capable of interpreting the profession of the prescribing physician. According to literature provided by Eicka and Reed (2000), once a drug receives approval by the United States Food and Drug Administration (USFDA) any physician may prescribe the medication for any indication and any age group the physician deems appropriate. This means that a podiatrist can prescribe an anti-psychotic to a toddler if it is deemed appropriate. The USFDA has made strides in attempting to provide and enforce legislative regulations for ensuring the availability of safety data and recommendations for medications used in children. Eicka and Reed (2000) further cite that The Final Rule, which became effective in 1999, provides incentives (and penalties) to those manufacturers that make data available. However, "off-label" prescribing remains legal as long as warnings of unknown risks toward children are marked on the label.

Zima et al. (1999) did not examine prescribed medications other than stimulants in relationship to the given diagnosis. This data is key in determining the efficacy of prescribed medications when prescribing for "off-label" purposes. For example, Cooper, Federspiel, Griffin, and Hickson (1998) found that a large proportion of children on the Tennessee Medicaid program were prescribed anti-convulsants for reasons other than seizures or epilepsy. The efficacy and safety of such medications used for alternate treatments is unknown and poses concern.

Trends in prescribing psychotropic medications to children and adolescents show that such use has increased over time (Zito et al., 2000). Zito et al. (2000) have also argued that "off-label" prescribing practices are common among physicians with or without psychiatric training. What has not been established are the long-term effects of safety and efficacy that commonly prescribed "off-label" medications can have on children and adolescents.

Even with these concerns in regard to pharmacotherapy practices in general, it is more disconcerting that little is known about the frequency and types of medication used with children and youth in foster care as well as the medication practices of the professionals involved. The primary purpose of this study was to examine the type and frequency of medication of all children and youth in the foster care system in a south Florida county for April 2001.

METHODS

The sample consisted of all children and youth in the foster care system during April, 2001 in a south Florida county. Of the 722 foster care youth in the total sample, 159 children (23%) were currently on prescribed medication. These 159 children, the medication sample, will be the primary focus of this investigation. However, comparisons to other children not currently using medication (n = 563, 88%) will be included for examining potential differences between the two groups.

Case file reviews were conducted on all 722 subjects. Training sessions were held with research assistants to establish a level of .95 inter-rater reliability. In addition, structured interviews with targeted case managers were also conducted for the medication sample only (n = 159).

RESULTS

Socio-Demographic Characteristics of Medication Sample

Of the 159 foster children and youth currently receiving medication, more than half the sample (56%) were male and also between the ages of 13 and 18 years (52%) (see Table 1). Forty-one percent were between the ages of 6 and 12 years. In terms of race, almost half (49%) were white, while 42% were black.

Medications Prescribed

Of the total sample of 722 cases, 23% (n = 201) were currently found to be on medication (see Table 2). The most frequently prescribed medications in ranked order were: the anti-psychotic drug Risperdal (4% of total sample, n = 30), Clonidine (3%, n = 21), Adderall (3%, n = 20), Ritalin (3%, n = 19), Depacote (3%, n = 19), Concerta (3%, n = 14), Phengram (3%, n = 13), Zyprexa (2%, n = 11), Paxil (2%, n = 11), Zoloft (2%, n = 11), Trazodone (1%, n = 8), Prozac (1%, n = 7), Impramine (1%, n = 7), and Wellbutrin (< 1%, n = 6). The majority of subjects had multiple prescriptions (57%) while 43% had one or a single

TABLE 1. Socio-Demographic Characteristics of Sample: Medication and No Medication

	On Medication (n = 159)		No Medication (n = 563)	
Gender	n	%	n	%
Female	70	44	263	47
Male	89	56	300	53
Age (years)				
0-5	9	6	168	30
6-12	65	41	184	33
13-18	83	52	174	31
19 and above	2	1	37	7
Race				
White	78	48	303	54
Black	66	42	211	38
Hispanic	10	6	23	4
Asian	1	< 1	10	2
Others	5	3	16	3

TABLE 2. Frequency of Medications Prescribed for Foster Care: Top 15

	Current Use*		Past Use*		Both*	
Medication	n	%	n	%	n	%
Risperdal	30	4	15	2	13	2
Clonidine	21	3	13	2	3	< 1
Adderall	20	3	9	1	9	1
Ritalin	19	3	23	5	9	1
Depacote	19	3	11	2	4	< 1
Concerta	14	3	1	< 1	0	0
Phengram	13	3	0	0	0	0
Neurontin	12	2	1	< 1	1	< 1
Zyprexa	11	2	9	1	2	< 1
Paxil	11	2	1	< 1	0	0
Zoloft	11	2	8	1	5	< 1
Trazodone	8	1	4	1	0	0
Prozac	7	1	18	4	4	< 1
Impramine	7	1	6	1	3	< 1
Wellbutrin	6	< 1	9	1	2	< 1

*% of total sample (n = 722)

prescription. Finally, all possible permutations of the different possible multiple drugs were examined and no frequent pattern was found.

The most frequent behaviors and symptoms found were sadness (17%, n = 35), delinquency history (13%, n = 26), and argumentative behavior (11%, n = 21) (see Table 3). Behaviors accounting for ten percent or less each were "easily angered," " running away," "impulsive," "aggressive," "anxious," "fearful," "stealing," "defiant," "easily distracted," and "restless."

Medication Practices of Professionals

Almost three-fourths (74%) of subjects had medications monitored while approximately a third did not have monitoring or there was no record in the files for monitoring (see Table 4). The most frequent schedule of monitoring of medication was monthly (48%) while the foster care placement (42%) was most likely to monitor medication. Finally, almost all prescribing of medications for foster care children and youth was done by psychiatrists (94%).

Foster Care Related

The most frequent placement for foster children and youth receiving medication was therapeutic foster care (28%), followed by foster home

TABLE 3. Most Frequent Behaviors/Symptoms Found for Prescription (Medication Sample Only)

Behaviors/Symptoms	On Medication		No Medication	
	n	%	n	%
Sad	35	17	59	13
Delinquency History	26	13	24	5
Argumentative	21	11	24	5
Easily Angered	20	10	3	9
Runs Away	20	10	34	7
Impulsive	20	10	25	5
Steals	18	9	24	6
Aggressive	17	9	54	11
Anxious/Fearful	17	9	48	9
Defiant	15	8	41	8
Easily Distracted	14	7	19	4
Restless	13	7	21	4

TABLE 4. Medication Practices of Professionals (Medication Sample Only)

	n	%
Medication was monitored		
Yes	102	64
No	57	36
Frequency of Monitoring		
Monthly	77	48
Quarterly	14	9
Weekly	4	3
Other	7	3
None	57	36
Who Monitors Medication?		
Placement	67	42
Case Manager	16	10
Health Professional	9	6
Foster Parent	8	5
Parent	8	5
Relative	5	3
School	4	3
None	42	26
Who Prescribes?		
Psychiatrist	148	94
Pediatrician	7	3
Other	4	2

(23%), residential group home (18%), placement with either a relative or non-relative (18%), and with a parent (9%) (see Table 5).

Mental Health

In terms of receiving a mental health evaluation, the sample was evenly divided on receiving either a psychological (56%) or a psychiatric evaluation (44%). The most frequent DSM-IV diagnoses were ADHD (20%), PTSD (10%), Major Depression (8%), and Bi-Polar Disorder (8%) (see Table 6). Of the total sample (n = 722), nine percent or 67 cases had been Baker Acted. In one of the most striking comparisons between the medication and no medication sample, 62 cases or 93% of those Baker Acted were currently on medication compared to only 5 cases for the non-medication sample.

Barriers to Services

Overall, few barriers to services (8%) were found for those receiving medication. Of those 22 cases reporting barriers, six were child refusals,

TABLE 5. Type of Foster Care Placement

	On Medication		No Medication	
	n	%	n	%
Therapeutic Foster Home	44	28	9	2
Foster Home	36	23	235	42
Residential Group Home	29	18	27	5
Relatives/Non	13	8	84	15
Parents	14	9	98	17
Other	5	3	21	4
Med Foster	6	4	20	4
Runaway	1	< 1	18	3
DJJ	6	4	13	2
Shelter	3	2	13	2

TABLE 6. Mental Health of Medicated Children and Youth in Foster Care

	On Medication		No Medication	
	n	%	n	%
Ever Baker Acted?	55	35	12	2
Yes	104	65	551	98
No				
DSM Diagnosis				
ADHD	31	20	11	2
Major Depression	12	8	24	4
PTSD	15	10	11	2
Bi-Polar Disorder	14	9	1	< 1
Victim of Neglect	10	6	45	8
Adjustment Disorder (emotion)	4	3	22	4
Dysthymia	5	3	3	< 1
Conduct Disorder	4	3	7	1
Adjustment Disorder (anxiety)	5	3	6	1
Intermittent Explosive	5	3	1	< 1
Oppositional Defiant	2	1	5	1
Adjustment Disorder (depression)	1	< 1	8	1

five were placed out of county, three were parent refusals, two were multiple placements, two were transportation difficulties, two were on waiting list, one moved out of the county, and one was runaway.

DISCUSSION

There were several concerns raised from this study on medication practices of children and adolescents in foster care. First was the finding that the most frequent drug prescribed was the adult anti-psychotic drug Risperdal. The use of this drug is of major concern given that it has not been tested for children and adolescents. This finding also begs the question of what standards exist to prescribe drugs to our youth. Furthermore, another concern was the majority of the medication sample had multiple rather than single prescriptions. Again, have such interactions been examined for youth and have such medications been tested for youth rather than just adults? Finally, there were a high number of foster youth on medication. One out of five foster care youth were on medication.

There were some positive findings on medication practices in foster care. First, few barriers to services were found. This possibly could be explained by reimbursement procedures that provide the incentive to those offering services to remove barriers. Next, there was some evidence of an appropriate service delivery match as individuals who receive medication also received more intense foster placements. This seems appropriate given the increased demands by those on medications such as monitoring, compliance with taking medication, and side-effects, etc.

Another finding of interest was that the medication sample was much more likely to have been previously Baker Acted. It would seem logical this finding is a result that more psychiatric disorders are indeed present in the individual and hence more medication is needed in the future. From a treatment perspective, however, this could be a time to conduct intensive intervention to determine if medication could be prevented in the future, relying more on, for example, psychosocial coping skills instead. Further research is needed in this area.

Finally, several of the findings would indicate the possible need for the treatment of depression in this sample. First, the most frequent emotion reported by the medication and the non-medication sample was sadness. Secondly, DSM-IV diagnoses related to depression accounted for 20% of the medication sample. This is much lower than the rates for depression related disorders found in the non-medication sample and in the general population of children and adolescents as well. Further research is needed in this area to indeed confirm that depression is a factor in relation to those children and youth on medication in foster care. One major limitation for the present study was the reliance on file reviews for obtaining data for this study. The file reviews may have inaccuracies due to such issues as time lags or personal error.

REFERENCES

Bhatara, V., Kallepalli, R., Misra, L., & Awadallah, S. (1996). A possible clonidine-trazodone-dextramphetamine interaction in a 12-year-old boy. *Journal of Child & Adolescent Psychopharmacology, 65,* 203-209.

Cantwell, D., Swanson, J., & Connor, D. (1997). Case study: Adverse response to clonidine. *Journal of the American Academy of Child and Adolescent Psychiatry, 36,* 539-554.

Cohena, J., Mannarinoa, A., & Rogalb, S. (2001). Treatment practices for childhood posttraumatic stress disorder. *Child Abuse & Neglect, 25*(1), 123-135.

Cooper, W., Federspiel, C., Griffin, M., & Hickson, G. (1998). New use of anti-convulsant medications among children enrolled in the Tennessee Medicaid program. *Archives of Pediatrics and Adolescent Medicine, 151*(12), 1242-1246.

Diller, L. (2000). Are stimulants overprescribed? *Journal of the American Academy of Child and Adolescent Psychiatry, 39*(3), 269.

Eicka, A., & Reed, M. (2000). Clinical pharmacology research in the pediatric patient: The challenge continues. *Progress in Pediatric Cardiology, 12*(1), 29-35.

Fenicel, R. (1995). Combining methylphenidate and clonidine: The role of post marketing surveillance. *Journal of Child and Adolescent Psychopharmacology, 5,* 155-156.

Geller, B., Reising, D., & Leonard, H. (1999). Critical review of tricyclic antidepressant use in children and adolescents. *Journal of the American Academy of Child and Adolescent Psychiatry, 38*(5), 513-516.

Hoar, W. (1998). Prozac Rx for children jumps 500%. *Mental Health News Alert, Sept. 29,* 13.

Jensen, P., Bhatara, V., & Vitiello, B. (1999). Psychoactive medication prescribing practices for U.S. children: Gaps between research and clinical practice. *Journal of the American Academy of Child and Adolescent Psychiatry, 38*(5), 557-565.

Journal of the American Academy of Child and Adolescent Psychiatry. (1999). Special Section: Current knowledge and unmet needs in pediatric psychopharmacology. Author: *38*(5), 501-565.

Leslie, L., Landsverk, J., Ezzet-Lofstrom, R., Tschann, J., Slymen, D., & Garland, A. (2000). Children in foster care: Factors influencing outpatient mental health service use. *Child Abuse & Neglect, 24*(4), 465-476.

Popper, C., & Zimnitzky, B. (1995). Sudden death putatively related to desipramine treatment in youth: A fifth case and review of speculative mechanisms. *Journal of Child and Adolescent Psychopharmacology, 5,* 283-300.

Storch, D. (1998). Outpatient pharmacotherapy in a community mental health center. *Journal of the American Academy of Child and Adolescent Psychiatry, 37*(3), 249-250.

Takayama, J., Bergman, A., & Connell, F. (1994). Children in foster care in the state of Washington: Health care utilization and expenditures. *Journal of the American Medical Association, 271,* 1850-1855.

University of North Carolina at Chapel Hill School of Medicine. (1999). Newest depression medications widely prescribed for children [On-line]. Available: *http://www.sciencedaily.com/releases/1999/05/990503041727.htm*

Vitiello, B., Jensen, P., & Hoagwooda, K. (1999). Integrating science and ethics in child and adolescent psychiatry research. *Biological Psychiatry, 46*(8), 1044-1049.

Walkup, J., Labellarte, M., & Riddle, M. (1998). Commentary: Unmasked and uncontrolled medication trials in child and adolescent psychiatry. *Journal of the American Academy of Child and Adolescent Psychiatry, 37*(4), 360-363.

Wilens, T., Biederman, J., Mick, E., & Spencer, T. (1995). A systematic assessment of tricyclic antidepressants in the treatment of adult attention deficit hyperactivity disorder. *Journal of Nerve Mental Disorders, 183*, 48-50.

Woolston, J. (1999). Combined pharmacotherapy: Pitfalls of treatment. *Journal of the American Academy of Child and Adolescent Psychiatry, 38*(11), 1455-1457.

Zima, B., Bussing, R., & Crecelius, G. (1999). Psychotropic medication use among children in foster care: Relationship to severe psychiatric disorders. *American Journal of Public Health, 89*(11), 1732-1735.

Zito, J., Safer, D., dosReis, S., Gardner, J., Boles, M., & Lynch, F. (2000). Trends in the prescribing of psychotropic medications to preschoolers. *The Journal of the American Medical Association, 283*(8), 1025-1030.

Attention-Deficit/Hyperactivity Disorder in Community College Students: A Seldom Considered Factor in Academic Success

Paula Gilbert

SUMMARY. Attention-Deficit/Hyperactivity Disorder (ADHD) is often unrecognized and infrequently treated in community college students. Since students with disabilities including ADHD are more likely to attend a 2-year rather than a 4-year college and to drop out before graduating, this article describes current conceptualizations of adult ADHD for community college social workers, psychologists, faculty, counselors, and staff. It presents counseling and educational interventions, which can result in greater academic success and an increase in self-esteem for individual students, as well as an increase in retention rates for the college. *[Article copies available for a fee from The Haworth Document Delivery Service: 1-800-HAWORTH. E-mail address: <docdelivery@haworthpress.com> Website: <http://www.HaworthPress.com> © 2005 by The Haworth Press, Inc. All rights reserved.]*

Paula Gilbert, MA, MSW, CSW, is affiliated with Psychological Services, Department of Student Development, Bronx Community College, City University of New York, Bronx NY 10453.

[Haworth co-indexing entry note]: "Attention-Deficit/Hyperactivity Disorder in Community College Students: A Seldom Considered Factor in Academic Success." Gilbert, Paula. Co-published simultaneously in *Journal of Social Work in Disability & Rehabilitation* (The Haworth Social Work Practice Press, an imprint of The Haworth Press, Inc.) Vol. 4, No. 1/2, 2005, pp. 57-75; and: *Disability Issues for Social Workers and Human Services Professionals in the Twenty-First Century* (ed: John W. Murphy, and John T. Pardeck) The Haworth Social Work Practice Press, an imprint of The Haworth Press, Inc., 2005, pp. 57-75. Single or multiple copies of this article are available for a fee from The Haworth Document Delivery Service [1-800-HAWORTH, 9:00 a.m. - 5:00 p.m. (EST). E-mail address: docdelivery@haworthpress.com].

Digital Object Identifier: 10.1300/J198v04n01_04

KEYWORDS. Attention-deficit/hyperactivity disorder, attention-deficit disorder, ADHD, ADD, community college students, disabilities

Attention-Deficit/Hyperactivity Disorder (ADHD)[1] can be a factor in exacerbating difficulties that community college students, often ranging in age from 18 to 50, may have in trying to succeed academically and to remain in college. Many with ADHD feel frustrated with unidentified learning difficulties or performance problems and suffer from low self-esteem, which may be factors contributing to their decisions about whether or not to stay in college.

This disorder, a discrete psychiatric and neurological phenomenon, has generally been diagnosed as a childhood condition. In the past few years, however, there have been studies to indicate that symptoms of ADHD may persist into adulthood for 50 to 65 percent of those having the disorder in childhood (Barkley, 1998). This comprises approximately two to six percent of the adult population (Weiss & Murray, 2003). While there appear to be few empirical statistics to determine the number of four year or two year college students with ADHD, DuPaul et al. (2001), examining self-reports of a sample of students from the United States, Italy and New Zealand, estimate that 2.9 to 8.1 percent of university students have ADHD, and Farrell (2003) suggests that from 0.5 to five percent of all college students have ADHD. It would not be unreasonable, therefore, to assume that one to four percent of community college students might have ADHD, causing difficulties in academic progress and that one to three percent of community college students would be likely to withdraw without completing a degree, if they do not have access to sufficient supportive services to address their condition. Moreover, since the National Center for Education Statistics (2000) reports that seven percent of students with a disability in two-year public colleges attain an Associate's degree compared to 18 percent of students without a disability, assisting students with ADHD and other disorders could be significant in terms of college retention.

Wolf (2001) indicates that adult students with ADHD may have difficulties because of "persistent cognitive deficits, deficiencies in basic skills, poor use of study strategies including organization and time management, lack of appropriate social skills, and low self-esteem" (p. 387). She points out that:

> Students with disabilities are more likely to pursue two-year versus four-year degrees and to drop out of college prior to complet-

ing a degree . . . Vulnerability is seen in the first two years, with notable difficulty in transition from secondary to postsecondary settings, particularly among young people with LD [learning disorders], ADHD, and psychiatric disorders . . . Once in college, students with disabilities may require more remedial or skills-level courses to maintain enrollment and may take longer to attain a degree or certificate. Nearly half of all disabled students drop out, compared with one-third of students without disabilities. The dropout rate climbs to nearly two-thirds for students with learning disabilities or "other" [including ADHD and psychiatric] disabilities. (p. 387)

In spite of the above statements that individuals with ADHD would be more likely to enter two-year schools and could be expected to have difficulties with academic work, few articles have been written about ADHD and community college students. Moreover, Glutting, Monaghan, Adams, and Sheslow (2002) reported that no prospective studies of college students with ADHD have been undertaken with investigation of the condition's onset, course, or treatment. Community college social workers, psychologists, counselors, faculty and staff need to become more aware of characteristics of adults with ADHD and work to provide appropriate teaching, learning and testing environments, supportive services, and where necessary, outside referrals for students with the disorder. If students with ADHD can receive these kinds of services, more should be able to remain in their community college, rather than withdrawing.

RECOGNIZING ADULT ADHD

The Diagnostic and Statistical Manual of Mental Disorders (Fourth Edition-Text Revision) (DSM-IV-TR), published by the American Psychiatric Association (APA) (2002), delineates diagnostic criteria for Attention-Deficit/Hyperactivity Disorder (ADHD). It is a condition usually first diagnosed or apparent in childhood, when individuals may have symptoms predominantly of inattention or of hyperactivity-impulsivity or a combination of both. The symptoms generally appear in home, school, work or social situations. DSM-IV-TR currently lists the same criteria for a diagnosis of ADHD in children and adults: six or more criteria for inattention and six or more criteria for hyperactivity-impulsivity. However, adults may exhibit fewer criteria. DSM-IV-TR indicates that symptoms, particularly of hyperactivity, lessen during late adolescence and adulthood for most individuals, although some experience the full complement of symptoms, especially of inattention, into mid-adulthood. In adult college students, problems with inattention are seen to become more prevalent, particularly as increasing numbers of women, whose inattention was not noticed when they were younger, are newly diagnosed with the disorder (Ratey, Miller, & Nadeau, 1995).

Those who have problems with attentiveness may not give close attention to details, may make careless mistakes in schoolwork and have difficulty concentrating on material. They may be distractible, i.e., very aware of background noises or visual stimuli. Students who have disorganization problems may be unable to complete tasks or to structure time; they may often lose things. Individuals with problems of impulsivity tend to act first and think second; they may interrupt while others speak, or be constantly on the go. DSM-IV-TR indicates that symptoms of hyperactivity in adults take the form of feelings of restlessness and problems with engaging in sedentary activities, which may lead a person to have difficulty both in sitting in classes and in doing homework. To be diagnosed with ADHD, an adult needs to have experienced symptoms of impairment before age seven (which may be determined at a later age through a retrospective history study and analysis) and the symptoms need to be present in two or more settings: at school, work, home or socially.

The diagnostic criteria contained in DSM-IV-TR, a compilation of the results of field studies and work by many psychiatric teams, contains most of the current criteria and descriptors of ADHD. It is important to note, however, that descriptions of diagnoses may change over time as more studies are undertaken to further knowledge about psychiatric conditions. The following descriptions by researchers who have been studying the underlying symptoms and mechanisms in adult ADHD help explain and further describe the condition.

Barkley (1997b) indicates that individuals with ADHD, primarily hyperactive and combined types, have difficulty with behavioral inhibition. He says they have behavior that is "less internally guided, less purposeful, less goal directed, less governed by and oriented to time, and less likely to be aimed at maximizing net future outcomes in lieu of immediate ones" (p. 277). Barkley (1998) also reports that adults with ADHD may have problems with: (1) remembering to do things, i.e., they may have problems with sense of and use of time, especially with regard to notions of hindsight and foresight since they think primarily of the temporal now; (2) separating the emotional aspects of a situation from the informational content; (3) being able to use internal language to guide behavior; and (4) being able to analyze problem situations, e.g., breaking the task or problem into component parts and being able to recombine or reconstitute the parts to come up with creative solutions, while maintaining flexibility in pursuing long term goals. Pennington (1991) states that ADHD has been interpreted as possibly resulting in faulty inhibitory mechanisms as well as decreased abilities in executive functioning– "an ability to maintain an appropriate problem-solving set for attainment of a future goal" (p. 13)–which refers to planning, organizational processes, and selective attention, as well as inhibitory control and creativity.

Mirsky (1996) focuses on attentional difficulties of those with ADHD. He indicates that attention is a complex set of four or five processes that may be distinct, but allow for shared responsibility. *Focusing/executing* refers to the "capacity to concentrate attention resources . . . on a specific task and to be able to screen out distracting peripheral stimuli," while *sustaining* "entails being able to stay on task in a vigilant manner for an appreciable interval" (Mirsky, 1996, pp. 76-77). In addition, *shifting* describes the capacity to change focus in an efficient manner, *stabilizing* requires reliability or consistency of attentional effort, and *encoding* involves "holding information briefly in mind while performing some action or cognitive operation upon it" (Mirsky, 1996, pp. 76-77).

Brown's (1996) research focuses primarily on the inattentive, cognitive and affective problems of those with ADHD including some aspects not described in DSM-IV-TR. He reports that adults with ADHD have problems with memory, and describes difficulties that they have in getting started, in maintaining effort for tasks, and in managing affective interference including problems with mood and sensitivity to criticism.

Social workers, psychologists, faculty, counselors, and staff at community colleges may recognize several of the behavioral and cognitive manifestations and symptoms of adult ADHD described above. Connecting and interrelating these symptoms and explanations can be useful in understanding ADHD and in helping students manage and deal with their disorder.

POSSIBLE CAUSES OF ADHD

In spite of extensive research efforts, the etiology of the disorder has not been definitively established. It is known, however, that genetic factors have been implicated in the condition for more than 50% of those with ADHD. According to Pauls (1991), identical twins are more likely to exhibit ADHD than fraternal twins and siblings of children with ADHD are twice as likely to have the disorder as would the general population. Biederman et al. (1995) studied increased risks of individuals inheriting ADHD from their biological parents. Furthermore, both neurological damage and physical trauma may also be the cause of the disorder; however, psychological trauma is generally considered to be an exacerbating condition and environmental or psychosocial factors such as school quality and family life can affect outcomes positively or negatively (Barkley, 1997a).

For the last several years, researchers have studied how brain chemistry and possible under-activity of several portions of the brain, primarily but not exclusively the frontal lobe, may result in an individual's having symptoms of ADHD. Since stimulants and/or some antidepressants have been shown to reduce symptoms of the disorder, researchers have also focused their studies on neurochemical functioning of the brain. Stefanatos and Wasserstein (2001) reported that ADHD may be a syndrome of the right hemisphere of the brain, and Giedd, Blumenthal, Molloy, and Castellanos (2001), who undertook studies utilizing positron emission tomography (PET), have found decreased blood flow and lower metabolic rates in the frontal lobe areas of children with ADHD and, in some cases, decreased size in portions of the brain as compared with controls.

POSSIBLE CO-EXISTING CONDITIONS

There have been many studies that look at co-existing or co-morbid conditions of those with ADHD. Twin and other studies indicate that Attention-Deficit Disorder and learning disabilities are independent conditions, transmitted independently, but that there is a significant cross-concordance between the two conditions (Faraone et al., 1993). It has been estimated that between 25 and 34 percent of students with ADHD also have learning disabilities (Byron & Parker, 2002). Reporting on results of several studies, Wilens et al. (2001) indicate that adults with ADHD have high rates of academic and occupational underachievement, social dysfunction, and psychopathology (particularly conduct and oppositional defiant disorders with associated antisocial acts and aggressiveness); moreover, many adults being treated for depression and substance abuse also have ADHD. The substance abuse may be the result of impulsivity or conduct disorder or a type of self-medication, where the student tries to feel better, e.g., to have greater self-esteem and less anxiety, especially when his or her ADHD is untreated (Kilcarr, 1998). Several researchers have indicated that childhood treatment of ADHD with stimulants does not increase the likelihood of adult abuse of stimulants.

There is no question that the variations in the descriptions of co-morbid conditions make accurate diagnosing of ADHD more difficult. However, when co-existing conditions are identified with ADHD, it is important to treat the other condition or conditions, e.g., substance abuse, depression, learning disorders, as well as the attention disorder. As discussed later, these variations may also aid in understanding differences in responses to clinical courses and pharmaco-therapeutic interventions. For example, some individuals may respond positively to stimulant medications, while others may respond better to antidepressants or mood stabilizers. Equally importantly, some psychological difficulties, such as depression, may be the result of an individual's reaction to living with some of the various undermining characteristics of ADHD.

ADHD IN COMMUNITY COLLEGE STUDENTS

Community college students with ADHD may exhibit problems with inattention, cognitive processes, impulsivity or restlessness. They may be inefficient in terms of planning and using time and resources; they would be likely to have difficulty sitting in classes, reading, studying, writing papers, and taking exams. They may have difficulty concentrating, may not give close attention to detail and may make careless mistakes in schoolwork or struggle with problems of memory or thinking. In addition, they may find it hard to plan and use time in an organized way, and to begin or stay with assignments and finish them, especially assignments that are long and/or that have a due date later in the semester. They may appear fidgety, moving hands or feet frequently or squirming in their seats. They may also blurt out answers, unable to wait their turn or listen to the full question being asked.

Having ADHD may be compared to trying to run a race while carrying a backpack full of stones; one may finish the race and may even win it, but the amount of energy that an individual needs to expend to do so is generally significantly greater than that of the other people running or completing that task. Educators need to help these students lighten their loads, gain knowledge about their disorder and reframe their outlooks.

HELP AT THE COMMUNITY COLLEGE

Adult ADHD is a disorder affecting many parts of an individual's life and it can be particularly disruptive to a student's academic ambitions. It is a condition that cannot be cured, but one that can be understood and managed or reduced in impact. If community college students with this disorder can get some assistance, they can generally succeed in their academic pursuits. As Wolf (2001) points out, "support systems become particularly important in providing . . . [the ADD] student with navigational skills to overcome these obstacles" (p. 388). Moreover, the supports and skill-building efforts should be designed to foster growth, self-management, self-determination, independence, and confidence in students with ADHD.

Community college faculty, psychologists, social workers, disabilities professionals, health professionals, and some others on the community college campus can undertake approaches and techniques described in the following sections. Alternatively, these individuals may be able to refer students off-campus for some of the services. Wherever possible, it is desirable to form a team of student support professionals, together with faculty and tutors and individuals acting as coaches, to develop networks for assisting adult students with ADHD. A social worker, psychologist, disabilities specialist or counselor, who is aware of the students' needs and of helping systems to address those needs and can monitor the students' progress, could be the head of the community college team for each student or small group of students. Administrators need to be aware of the disorder so that they can create appropriate policies and can support efforts undertaken by faculty and staff assisting students.

The approaches/techniques that can be used at the community college include: Identification of students with the disorder, education about adult ADHD, counseling, teaching techniques, remedial classes, coaching, therapy, tutoring, helping with understanding the use of medication, and providing accommodations relating to disability regulations. It is important to note that for treating or ameliorating ADHD symptoms, it is generally effective and desirable to use two or more modalities. It is also important to remember that whatever approaches and/or techniques are utilized, the goal is empowerment of the student.

Identification

Faculty, counselors, disability specialists, psychologists, social workers and tutors at learning centers, tutoring centers, skills building centers, and reading and writing labs should be on the lookout for students in class, in counseling sessions or getting services who have difficulties with reading and writing skills or who are having significant academic difficulty, e.g., failing courses or having a probation status. If no co-existing conditions or other explanations for the difficulties are apparent, they should also inquire about or listen for whether or not these students have problems with time management, focusing or organizational skills, as well as interpersonal or employment problems, i.e., difficulty with maintaining jobs and relationships. For example, when asked, students with ADHD may report being repeatedly late for classes and other appointments, and/or have a series of impulsivity-related experiences, such as several automobile accidents. Some students with ADHD may seem to be lazy, not trying hard enough, functioning erratically or displaying work of inconsistent quality.

A community college student having academic difficulties with the above characteristics should be referred to a social worker, psychologist or disability professional to evaluate that individual's symptoms and behaviors. Students with learning disorders or mental disorders such as depression or generalized anxiety may also have ADHD. In addition, as mentioned above, some students with undiagnosed ADHD may respond to academic and social pressure by self-medicating, that is, turning to alcohol or drugs to try to ease pressures that they feel. For diagnosis of the individual student, the mental health and disability professionals may be able to interview students on campus or provide referrals to an outside agency or an individual professional.

At the present time, a diagnosis of ADHD is established by a social worker, psychologist, psychiatrist, neurologist, or neuropsychologist, through the use of interviews, checklists, and rating scales. These professionals also can gather a thorough history of an individual's behavior over time, because the "story" told by the individual (self-report) and by his or her family or household members, if possible, is very important. Many practitioners use or modify the Utah Criteria for the Diagnosis of ADD Residual Type or the Utah Rating Scale prepared by Wender and his colleagues at the University of Utah Medical School (Wender, 2000) for a retrospective diagnosis. Some utilize a series of questions about an individual's developmental, employment, and health (including psychiatric) histories, as well as interview questions for that individual and his or her family members prepared by Barkley and co-workers at the University of Massachusetts Medical Center (Barkley & Murphy, 1998) and they combine these with symptom and performance rating scales. Others use the Brown ADD Scales (Brown, 1996) or Conners

Adult ADHD Rating Scale (Conners, Erhardt, & Sparrow, 1995). Neuropsychologists, other psychologists and some learning specialists may also administer aptitude, achievement, and information processing tests and other diagnostic materials before making recommendations for accommodations (Parker & Benedict, 2002).

Some college students have been identified as having ADHD at the elementary, middle, and high school levels and some have been receiving treatment and accommodations. The majority of community college students who are suffering from the disorder have not been identified before arriving at the campus.

Education About the Syndrome

It is important for students to learn more about adult ADHD through reading printed materials, viewing videos, listening to tapes, or conducting internet searches about the condition and asking questions individually or in groups. College social workers, psychologists, and disabilities professionals can provide pamphlets, show videos and conduct workshops and/or groups about the disorder. Students can also be informed about local and nationally supported groups, such as chapters of Children and Adults with Attention-Deficit Disorder (CHADD).

In the community college students may first be learning that they have ADHD or may be understanding better the implications and characteristics of the disorder, and what some of the possible deficits might be. However, while some or all of the terminology might be new for these students, the condition itself has undoubtedly been a source of disappointment and stress for them for many years, as they have felt unable to accomplish tasks as well as fellow students because of some combination of difficulties presented above. Knowledge about the disorder may be freeing, as students gain a better understanding of their experiences.

Social workers and psychologists can use workshop sessions or departmental meetings to help teaching faculty become more aware of the conceptualizations of adult students who may have ADHD. Follow-up sessions are important to give faculty an opportunity to present information, questions, and concerns.

Counseling

Social workers, psychologists, counselors, and others in support services can provide many types of assistance in individual or group formats. As Bramer (1996) points out, it is important that they "intervene with positive attitudes and affect" (p. 81). They can help with issues of time management (including procrastination or lateness), organization, problem-solving, and anger management. They can encourage students to focus on their strengths as well as on areas requiring assistance, especially in regard to choosing major concentrations or planning for a career or vocation. Social workers, psychologists, and counselors can also assist students with short-term goal setting, provide assistance with co-existing conditions such as depression and anxiety, teach stress reduction techniques, and the impact of ADHD on various aspects of their lives. They can remind students that it is not desirable to take on too many responsibilities or activities while in community college, but it can be helpful to get some physical exercise and to seek limited opportunities to socialize with other students.

While skill building and skill practicing are important for all community college students and are generally included in the curricula of freshmen orientation classes (often taught by counselors), they are continuing necessities for students with attention deficits. Counselors, disability specialists or others, acting as coaches, may provide on-going help. It is often beneficial to use a case management system in assisting community college students with ADHD, i.e., one counselor or disability specialist would have a caseload of students and work with them for many, if not all, semesters.

Adult students with ADHD generally benefit from vocational and career counseling to explore possible community college majors and concentrations, careers, employment fields, and types of jobs that might be suitable and interesting to them. As students learn and practice focusing on longer range thinking, they also need periodic help with academic advisement in terms of appropriate courses and course loads. In all cases, students should be encouraged to look at their strengths as well as their areas of difficulty.

Teaching

Since ADHD can be considered a condition of inadequate internal thought and regulation, it is helpful for faculty to externalize and make more explicit some of their own thought processes and organizational systems, which could be helpful to all students and especially to those with ADHD. Faculty can help students focus and keep more organized by clearly stating work to be assigned, emphasizing due dates, putting as much information as possible in writing–whether on the board, in handouts, on overhead slides or in power point outlines. They can teach in a structured, consistent manner, e.g., by providing some outlines of how different aspects of course content relate to one another and by explaining study strategies. It is also helpful if faculty review work from a prior session at the beginning of a class and summarize key points at the end of the current class. They can provide opportunities for students to tape lectures and to learn through multi-sensory techniques. It would also be desirable for faculty to break assignments and tasks into smaller components, and create shorter time interval requirements.

Remedial and/or Skill-Building Classes

Since many, although not all, community college students with ADHD have deficiencies in reading, writing and mathematics skills, it is helpful for them to have remedial or skill-building courses taught by academic faculty or support services providers. Counselors and mental health professionals can work with faculty to help students help themselves; students will benefit from learning and practicing note-taking, study skills, organization and time management strategies.

Barkley (1998) points out that sometimes individuals with ADHD know *what* to do, but do not know when or how to do things. By learning and practicing in a supportive, non-threatening environment, students may be better able to use their talents.

Coaching

Hallowell and Ratey (1994) have encouraged the use of coaching by those who are knowledgeable about ADHD and coaching techniques. This might include social workers, psychologists, faculty, counselors, tutors, partners and parents, as well as other individuals on or off campus. Modeled after coaching of individual athletic team members, this technique or process provides a combination of helping to establish goals and strategies for achieving the goals, reminding the student what he or she can do and when to do it, as well as supporting and encouraging that student.

Coaches may provide a support system and structure, whenever students change environments by going from high school, alternative programs, employment, or family commitments to the very different setting and requirements of a community college. Coaches for students with ADHD can help them identify and prioritize their own academic goals, and help them develop strategies and steps to achieve the goals.

Tutoring/Peer Counseling

Tutors, who generally provide assistance in subject area courses or help students with improving their reading and writing skills, are also very important to community college students with ADHD. Tutors may be staff, but are often successful students, as are peer counselors, who can provide encouragement through sharing first hand knowledge and experience. They may effectively discuss academic or personal issues with students. Since tutors and peer counselors may be found in many different locations and/or departments on a community college campus, it is important to include, if possible, combined or common training time for them devoted to recognizing, working with and referring students with ADHD.

Therapy

As a result of their life long experience of deficits in a few or many settings, most students with ADHD suffer from low self-esteem and frequent frustration. In addition, generally for reasons of genetics, self-image or socialization, many of these adult students suffer from some co-existing condition such as depression, anxiety or substance abuse. On or off campus mental health professionals can provide individual supportive psychotherapy and/or cognitive-behavioral therapy (CBT). It should be noted that both forms of therapy can share conceptual aspects of the other; they may be invaluable in assisting an individual to make changes in dealing with the disorder and in becoming more academically successful at the community college. Psychotherapy may help students deal with their feelings about their experience of academic, relationship and other personal problems, learn about alternate patterns of thinking and behaving, and increase self-esteem. Pliszka, Carlson, and Swanson (1999) consider CBT, which may involve reframing negative thoughts into positive statements and modifying problem behaviors by learning about and practicing new behaviors, to be very helpful, particularly in combination with medication. With CBT, for example, a student may learn how to break up assignments into smaller units, apply the practice to one or more course tasks, and set a reward for completing the process. In therapy groups, adults with ADHD can share thoughts, experiences and feelings, gain socializing experience, learn to manage and better deal with anger and frustration, and gain greater self-esteem.

Understanding Use of Medication

Community college health and mental health professionals can refer students with ADHD symptoms to psychiatrists for evaluations of their conditions and the suitability of medication. Wilens et al. (2001) report that psychiatrists most often prescribe the short acting stimulants or a combination of different forms of stimulants for longer effects, so that a student would not have to take doses during the school day. If stimulants are unsuitable or not tolerated, and particularly if depression is a co-morbid condition, psychiatrists often recommend one or a combination of antidepressants for adults with ADHD. Psychiatrists are very cautious about prescribing stimulants for individuals with a history of substance abuse (Wender, 2000). Where substance abuse has been a past problem, physicians have indicated that they would be more likely to utilize an antidepressant drug. Other conditions that may preclude the use of stimulants include Tourette's syndrome or anxiety. In some cases, especially where an individual has symptoms of aggression, mood stabilizers or anti-convulsants may be utilized (Goldstein & Goldstein, 1997). In most cases, social workers and psychologists on the campus can be very helpful in providing additional information about medications to help students make informed decisions.

Accommodations to Meet Legal Requirements

Students whose ADHD condition may qualify them as disabled, whether they have been identified while in the community college or in previous schools, are protected by and entitled to services under Section 504 of the Rehabilitation Act of 1973 (RA), as well as the Americans With Disabilities Act of 1990 (ADA). ADHD is considered a physical or mental condition, which may be at the level of a disability or substantial impairment. Latham and Latham (1997) indicate that:

> Individuals with ADD and specific LD [learning disabilities] are considered individuals with disabilities under federal law when their conditions are of sufficient severity to substantially limit a major life activity like learning or working. Individuals with these disabilities enjoy the right to be free from discrimination and to receive reasonable accommodations in the classroom and workplace under federal law. (p. 326)

Generally, documentation describing the student's impairments is based on the DSM checklist of criteria or other recognized inventories or checklists regarding current symptoms and historic information. It includes information about co-existing conditions including learning disabilities and psychological disorders, as well as suggested educational accommodations. Byron and Parker (2002) note that comprehensive evaluations including substantial historical material, consideration of possible co-existing disorders, and neuropsychological assessments are desirable.

Disability Services offices generally arrange for accommodations for students with ADHD which may include, among others: extended time for test taking; separate, quiet rooms for taking exams; readers; and/or note-takers. While some of these accommodations also may be used for students with learning or physical disabilities, accommodations in every case need to be tailored to meet the needs of the particular student.

CONCLUSIONS

We know that an adult student with ADHD cannot just "shape up and get the work done," but he or she can learn to use techniques to become more organized and to use time more effectively. Barkley (1998) reminds us that for adults with ADHD, "proper diagnosis, treatment, and motivation can make the difference between success and failure in school" (p. 583). It is anticipated that as diagnostic tools, treatment methods and support services improve and become more available, many of the adult community college students with ADHD will go from better understanding their limitations to better utilizing their strengths. In a similar vein, Bemporad (2001) states that through problem solving and other approaches, adults with ADHD will come to "regard themselves no longer as the helpless victim of uncontrollable forces but as the initiator and executor of desired goals" (p. 308).

Further research is needed concerning the prevalence of ADHD at the community college level, as well as the efficacy of methods used in colleges for identifying and assisting students in managing this disorder. Students come to community colleges with a very wide range of abilities and intelligence, vast differences in types and levels of high school or GED preparations, and significant differences in English language competencies, among other differences and variations along a broad continuum. In addition, many community college students are parents and/or hold full- or part-time jobs; the task of juggling multiple responsibilities is substantially harder for those with ADHD than for more typical students.

Faculty and staff in community colleges need to understand and remember that they can help students develop and practice strategies to overcome some of the students' functioning difficulties, and work with them on effectively organizing material and tasks and utilizing time. The experience of this type of support will go a long way toward boosting those students' self-esteem and hope, which in turn can lead to future successes. Murphy (1995) states that adults:

> . . . need to realize that ADD is a treatable condition. They need to understand that they have some power, control, and responsibility in how effectively they learn to manage it. Instilling hope, fostering . . . a belief that they are potent and can succeed, and demonstrating a sincere and ongoing commitment to helping . . . [them] work around their difficulties appear to be important and sometimes overlooked components of treatment. (p. 144)

ADHD is a disorder that can limit a student's achievement or make it more difficult for him or her to meet aspirations, but it does not preclude that student's accomplishment and academic success. Skillful intervention can help lighten the load for the individual with ADHD and allow the community college and the larger society to benefit from the expanded use of his or her talents and self-esteem. Significantly as well, community colleges can increase retention rates, as more students with ADHD are recognized and assisted in overcoming their handicaps and capitalizing on their strengths.

NOTE

1. ADHD, AD/HD, and ADD will be used interchangeably in this article. ADHD is the diagnostic category listed in DSM-IV-TR; however, some feel that ADD is more appropriate for adults with attention deficits.

REFERENCES

American Psychiatric Association. (2002). *Diagnostic and statistical manual of mental disorders* (4th edition-text revision) Washington, DC: Author.

Barkley, R. A. (1997a). *ADHD and the nature of self-control.* New York: Guilford Press.

Barkley, R. A. (1997b). Attention-deficit hyperactivity disorder, self-regulation, and time: Toward a more comprehensive theory. *Developmental and Behavioral Pediatrics, 18*(4), 271-279.

Barkley, R. A. (1998). *Attention-deficit hyperactivity disorder: A handbook for diagnosis and treatment* (2nd edition). New York: Guilford Press.

Barkley, R. A., & Murphy, K.R. (1998). *Attention-deficit hyperactivity disorder: A clinical workbook* (2nd edition). New York: Guilford Press.

Bemporad, J. (2001). Aspects of psychotherapy with adults with attention deficit disorder. In J. Wasserstein, L.E. Woolf, & F. F. LeFever (Eds.), *Adult attention deficit disorder: Brain mechanisms and life outcomes: Annals of the New York Academy of Sciences (vol. 931,* pp. 302-309). New York: New York Academy of Sciences.

Biederman, J., Faraone, S.V., Mick, E., Spencer, T., Wilens, T., Kiely, K., Guite, J. Ablon, J.S., Reed, E., & Warburton, R. (1995). High risk for attention-deficit/hyperactivity disorder among children of parents with childhood onset of the disorder: A pilot study. *American Journal of Psychiatry, 152,* 431-435.

Bramer, J.S. (1996). Serving college students with attention deficit/hyperactivity disorder. *Michigan Community College Journal: Research and Practice, 2*(2), 73-84.

Brown, T.E. (1996). *Brown attention-deficit disorder scales.* San Antonio: Psychological Corp.

Byron, J., & Parker, D.R. (2002). College students with ADHD: New challenges and directions. In L.C. Brinckerhoff, J.M. McGuire, & S.F. Shaw (Eds.), *Postsecondary education and transition for students with learning disabilities,* 2nd ed. (pp. 335-387). Austin, Texas: PRO-ED.

Conners, C.K., Erhardt, D., & Sparrow, E. (1995). Conners adult ADHD rating scale. North Tonowanda, NY: Multi-Health Systems.

DuPaul, G. J., Schaughency, E.A., Weyandt, L.L., Tripp, G., Kiesner, J., Ota, K., & Standish, H. (2001). Self-report of ADHD symptoms in university students: Cross-gender and cross-national prevalence. *Journal of Learning Disabilities, 34* (4), 370-379.

Faraone, S.V., Biederman, J., Lehman, B.K., Keenan, K., Norman, D., Seidman, L.J., Koldodny, R., Kraus, I., Perrin, J., & Chen, W. J. (1993). Evidence for the independent familial transmission of attention-deficit/hyperactivity disorder and learning disabilities: Results from a family genetic study. *American Journal of Psychiatry, 150*(6), 891-895.

Farrell, E. F. (2003). Paying attention to students who can't. *Chronicle of Higher Education, 50*(5), A50-51.

Giedd, J.N., Blumenthal, J., Molloy, E., & Castellanos, F.X. (2001). In J. Wasserstein, L.E. Woolf, & F. F. LeFever (Eds.), *Adult attention deficit disorder: Brain mechanisms and life outcomes: Annals of the New York Academy of Sciences (vol. 931,* pp. 33-49). New York: New York Academy of Sciences.

Glutting, J.J., Monaghan, M.C., Adams, W., & Sheslow, D. (2002). Some psychometric properties of a system to measure ADHD among college students: Factor pattern, reliability, and one-year predictive validity. *Measurement and Evaluation in Counseling and Development, 34*(4), 194-209.

Goldstein, S., & Goldstein, M. (1997). Drugs affecting learning, attention, and memory. In S. Goldstein, *Managing attention and learning disorders in late adolescence and adulthood: A guide for practitioners* (pp. 327-373). New York: John Wiley and Sons.

Hallowell, E. M., & Ratey, J.J. (1994). *Driven to distraction*. New York: Pantheon.

Kilcarr, P. J. (1998). Additional risks facing college students with AD/HD. In P. Quinn & A. McCormick (Eds.), *Re-thinking AD/HD: A guide for fostering success in students with AD/HD at the college level* (pp. 67-75). Bethesda, Maryland: Advantage Books.

Latham, P.H., & Latham, P. S. (1997). Legal rights. In S. Goldstein, *Managing attention and learning disorders in late adolescence and adulthood: A guide for practitioners* (pp. 315- 326). New York: John Wiley and Sons.

Mirsky, A.F. (1996). Disorders of attention: A neuropsychological perspective. In G.R. Lyon, & N.A. Krasnegor (Eds.), *Attention, memory, and executive function*. Baltimore: Paul H. Brooks Publishing Co.

Murphy, K. (1995). Empowering the adult with ADD. In K. G. Nadeau (Ed.), *A comprehensive guide to attention deficit disorder in adults: Research, diagnosis and treatment* (pp. 135- 145). New York: Brunner/Mazel.

National Center for Educational Statistics, U.S. Department of Education. (2000). Postsecondary students with disabilities: Enrollment, services, and persistence in *Stats in Brief* (NCES 2000-092). Jessup, MD: Education Publications Center.

Parker, D.R., & Benedict, K.B. (2002). Assessment and intervention: Promoting successful transitions for college students with ADHD. *Assessment for Effective Intervention, 27*(3), 3-24.

Pauls, D.L. (1991). Genetic factors in the expression of attention-deficit hyperactivity disorder. *Journal of Child and Adolescent Psychopharmacology, 1*(5), 353-360.

Pennington, B.F. (1991). *Diagnosing learning disorders*. New York: Guilford Press.

Pliszka, S.R., Carlson, C.L., & Swanson, J.M. (1999). *ADHD with comorbid disorders: Clinical assessment and management*. New York: Guilford Press.

Ratey, J.J., Miller, A.C., & Nadeau, K.G. (1995). Special diagnostic and treatment considerations in women with attention-deficit disorder. In K.G. Nadeau (Ed.), *A comprehensive guide to attention deficit disorder in adults: Research, diagnosis, and treatment* (pp. 260-283). New York: Brunner/Mazel.

Stefanatos, G.A., & Wasserstein, J. (2001). Attention deficit/hyperactivity disorder as a right hemisphere syndrome: Selective literature review and detailed neuropsychological case studies. In J. Wasserstein, L.E. Woolf, & F. F. LeFever (Eds.), *Adult attention deficit disorder: Brain mechanisms and life outcomes: Annals of the New York Academy of Sciences (vol. 931*, pp. 172-195). New York: New York Academy of Sciences.

Weiss, M., & Murray, C. (2003). Assessment and management of attention-deficit hyperactivity disorder in adults. *Canadian Medical Association Journal, 168*(6), 715-722.

Wender, P.H. (2000). *ADHD: Attention-deficit hyperactivity disorder in children and adults*. Oxford: Oxford University Press.

Wilens, T.E., Spencer, T.J., Biederman, J., Girard, K., Doyle, R., Prince, J, Polisner, D., Solhkhah, R., Comeau, S., Monuteaux, M.C., & Parekh, A. (2001). A controlled clinical trial of buproprion for attention-deficit/hyperactivity disorder in adults. *American Journal of Psychiatry, 158*(2), 282-288.

Wolf, L. E. (2001) College students with ADHD and other hidden disabilities: Outcomes and interventions. In J. Wasserstein, L.E. Wolf, & F. F. LeFever (Eds.), *Adult attention deficit disorder: Brain mechanisms and life outcomes: Annals of the New York Academy of Sciences (vol. 931*, pp. 385-395). New York: New York Academy of Sciences.

Using Children's Books
as an Approach
to Enhancing Our Understanding
of Disability

John T. Pardeck

SUMMARY. Children's books can be used as a tool for teaching about the unique needs of children with disabilities. This article offers strategies for using books as a medium for increasing our understanding about disability. In the article a disability is viewed as an aspect of cultural diversity. A list of children's books focusing on the topic of disability is offered. *[Article copies available for a fee from The Haworth Document Delivery Service: 1-800-HAWORTH. E-mail address: <docdelivery@haworthpress.com> Website: <http://www.HaworthPress.com> © 2005 by The Haworth Press, Inc. All rights reserved.]*

KEYWORDS. Bibliotherapy, children's literature, disabilities, fairy tales, fiction, non-fiction, self-help books, picture books

John T. Pardeck, PhD, LCSW, was formerly Professor of Social Work, School of Social Work, Southwest Missouri State University, Springfield, MO 65804. He is now deceased.

[Haworth co-indexing entry note]: "Using Children's Books as an Approach to Enhancing Our Understanding of Disability." Pardeck, John T. Co-published simultaneously in *Journal of Social Work in Disability & Rehabilitation* (The Haworth Social Work Practice Press, an imprint of The Haworth Press, Inc.) Vol. 4, No. 1/2, 2005, pp. 77-85; and: *Disability Issues for Social Workers and Human Services Professionals in the Twenty-First Century* (ed: John W. Murphy, and John T. Pardeck) The Haworth Social Work Practice Press, an imprint of The Haworth Press, Inc., 2005, pp. 77-85. Single or multiple copies of this article are available for a fee from The Haworth Document Delivery Service [1-800-HAWORTH, 9:00 a.m. - 5:00 p.m. (EST). E-mail address: docdelivery@haworthpress.com].

http://www.haworthpress.com/web/JSWDR
© 2005 by The Haworth Press, Inc. All rights reserved.
Digital Object Identifier: 10.1300/J198v04n01_05

Samuel Crothers created the term bibliotherapy in 1916. Furthermore, at the turn of the Twentieth Century, the American Library Association endorsed the creation of libraries for patients in hospitals and other therapeutic settings. Drs. Karl and William Menninger were the first significant therapists to use bibliotherapy in treatment in the 1940s. Caroline Shrodes (1949) conducted the first significant research on bibliotherapy in her dissertation. In the 1990s, Albert Ellis (1995) and Santrock, Minnett, and Campbell (1994) supported the effectiveness of bibliotherapy in the therapeutic process. Even though bibliotherapy is a relatively new therapeutic approach to social work, it has a rich history with a number of notable therapists who have endorsed its use.

Bibliotherapy means treatment through the use of books. Smith and Burkhalter (1987) and Starker (1988) conclude that books, both fiction and nonfiction, can be used as effective tools for not only dealing with emotional problems, but also as a medium for helping individuals deal with issues ranging from advice on child development to personal development. Bernstein (1989) concludes that everyone has used books in some shape or form to increase their understanding of themselves, others, and their culture. The goal of this paper is to present how bibliotherapy can be used as a tool for increasing one's understanding of disability. A number of annotated books are offered that teachers and other professionals will find useful as tools for helping children to understand and appreciate the notion of disabilities as a form of cultural diversity.

DEFINING BIBLIOTHERAPY

Bibliotherapy is a group of techniques for structuring interaction between a facilitator and participant based on mutual sharing of literature (McKinney, 1977; Pardeck and Pardeck, 1998). The use of books in treatment has been interpreted differently by psychologists, nurses, social workers, and others. Among these professionals, there is confusion in determining the dividing line between reading guidance and bibliotherapy (Pardeck, 1998).

Bibliotherapy has also been known by several names, including bibliocounseling, library therapeutics, biblioprophylaxis, tutorial group therapy, and literatherapy (Pardeck, 1998). *Webster's New Collegiate Dictionary* (1981, p. 25) defines bibliotherapy as "guidance in the solution of personal problems through directed reading." Even though there are a number of definitions for bibliotherapy, increasing numbers of professionals including counselors, psychologists, and psychiatrists are using this emerging treatment approach in practice (Pardeck and Pardeck, 1998).

Hynes and Wedl (1990) provide additional insight into the uses of bibliotherapy. They conclude that bibliotherapy can be understood as a technique that can be delineated into four different processes. These are as follows:

1. Developmental interactive bibliotherapy refers to the use of books in places like schools to promote growth and development.
2. Bibliotherapy can be understood as a solitary process that requires no therapeutic involvement.
3. Bibliotherapy can be seen as a clinical interactive process that involves a practitioner.
4. Bibliotherapy can be seen as a creative writing process used in treatment.

This paper will focus on bibliotherapy as a technique that can promote the growth and development of children in the area of cultural diversity and their understanding of disability.

MEDIUMS FOR CONDUCTING BIBLIOTHERAPY

Five kinds of mediums that may be used for conducting bibliotherapy with children. Each of these may be used as resources for helping children gain insight and appreciation of special needs children who are important part of cultural diversity (Pardeck and Pardeck, 1998).

Fiction

Works of fiction portraying a specific issue (i.e., children with disabilities) in story form are an excellent resource for bibliotherapy. Children can read and identify with fictional characters and develop empathy for their plight. If the child is old enough, he or she can develop insight and greater understanding about the unique problems that special needs children face. Obviously, fiction can also be used as a resource for helping children in general develop greater insight into individual problems that they may be facing (Pardeck, 1998).

Nonfiction

Nonfiction books are also available on numerous topics including disabilities. Nonfictional books are a good match for children seeking information about a particular topic (Pardeck, 1998). A child can develop insight into a given issue through nonfiction because this kind of literature often offers extremely accurate descriptions of problem. Morris-Vann (1979) suggest that it is extremely important for the person working with children in the area of cultural diversity to identify resources that accurately reflect this topic.

Self-Help Books

Children will also find self-help books to be extremely helpful for understanding important issues. The self-help book concept is relatively new in the area of children's literature. The helping person working with children must be particularly sensitive to finding self-help books that appropriately reflect a topic or issue (Pardeck, 1998).

Fairy Tales

Fairy tales are a favorite way for children to learn about how they can solve problems. Fairy tales give simple portrayals of the universal problems and fears that have confronted children for centuries. Fairy tales offer a way for children to use their vivid imaginations as a strategy for problem solving and for understanding issues. There are a number of traditional fairy tales that can be very helpful for providing insight into various disabilities (Pardeck, 1998).

Picture Books

This kind of bibliotherapy is designed for young children. Children of this age group love picture books that have few words but have many colorful pictures. Picture books often reflect the feelings and thoughts possessed by children about an issue; children can project their inner feelings and perceptions onto the books' characters. This process helps them reveal their own conflicts in a nonthreatening way. Picture books provide a safe outlet for young children to tell their own stories in both individual and group settings. There are a number of picture books available that focus on the topic of disabilities. Picture books can be an excellent medium for teaching about disabilities to children who have not mastered reading due to their intellectual development or simply enjoy pictures over words (Pardeck, 1998).

THE BIBLIOTHERAPEUTIC PROCESS

The bibliotherapeutic process consist of a series of distinct activities critical to using books as a strategy to enhance cultural diversity. These include the child's readiness, book selection, as well as the child actually reading the book. The bibliotherapeutic process also calls for meaningful follow-up activities. These activities are aimed at moving the child through the stages of the bibliotherapeutic process (Pardeck and Pardeck, 1998).

Readiness

Before proceeding with the bibliotherapeutic process, the helping person must consider an important factor–the child's readiness for bibliotherapy. Inappropriate timing may impede the process. Typically, the child is ready for the initiation of bibliotherapy when the following conditions have been met:

1. Rapport, trust, and confidence have been established between the helping person and the child.
2. The child and the helper have agreed to work together.
3. Preliminary exploration of the goals of bibliotherapy have occurred (Zaccaria and Moses, 1968).

Selection of Books

The helping person must consider several factors when identifying books for use in the bibliotherapeutic process. The most important factor is the issue to be worked on (Coleman and Ganong, 1990). Although books are available on virtually any topic, it is essential when using books aimed at promoting growth and development that the work contain believable characters and situations. The helping person must also know the child's interest and reading levels. One additional element in book selection is the book's form of publication. Alternative forms such as Braille, talking books (cassettes), and large print are available for special needs children. The practitioner may wish to use a paperback edition when working with older children (Pardeck and Pardeck, 1998).

Introducing the Book

When the child is ready for the bibliotherapeutic process to begin and book selection has been completed, the helping person's next concern is how to introduce the book to the child. Most practitioners feel that it is best to suggest books rather than to prescribe them; however, one may have to prescribe books for very young children (Griffin, 1984). Regardless of what strategy the helping person uses for introducing books to children, he or she must be familiar with the content of the books selected (Pardeck and Pardeck, 1998).

Follow-Up Strategies

Zaccaria and Moses (1968) conclude that most studies dealing with the use of books for growth and development enhancement suggest that the reading of a book must be accompanied by discussion. Numerous activities can be utilized by the helping person after a book has been read. These activities are appropriate for most children. Certain follow-up activities require a group setting. Pardeck and Pardeck (1998) outline how creative writing, art activities, discussion, and role playing can be used as strategies for follow-up activities when conducting bibliotherapy.

The helping person should, of course, keep in mind the child's reading preferences when selecting books (Pardeck and Pardeck, 1998). The helping person can adapt the activities to fit each child's needs; for example, a child who dislikes writing can use a tape recorder for the creative writing activities. Depending on the child's needs and the type of book used, the helping person may wish to suggest several follow-up activities from which the child can select one or more (Pardeck and Pardeck, 1998).

RECOMMENDED CHILDREN'S BOOKS ON DISABILITIES

The following books are recommended as tools for teaching about disability and disability culture (Pardeck and Musick, 2002).

Adams, Barbara. *Like It Is: Facts and Feelings About Handicap From Kids Who Know.* New York: Walker, 1979. This book presents children discussing their disabilities, and the problems that often accompany them. Included is a range of disabilities, from emotional to learning disabilities.

Aseltine, Lorraine. *I'm Deaf and It's Okay.* Nile, IL: Albert Whitman, 1986. A narrator describes the frustrations caused by his deafness and explains how he copes. The narrator's dilemma is presented in a realistic fashion and can be used as a starting point for discussion of disabilities.

Baker, Pamel J. *My First Book of Sign.* Washington, DC: Gallaude University Press, 1986. Children are pictured forming words in sign language by illustrations of words. A discussion of fingerspelling and general rules for signing arc presented.

Brandenberg, Franz. *Otto Is Different.* New York, Greenwillow, 1985. Otto is an octopus who feels he is different from other animal friends because he has eight arms. However, he discovers that having eight arms can sometimes be to his advantage.

Brown, Tricia. *Someone Special, Just Like You.* New York: Holt, Rinehart and Winston, 1984. This book offers black-and-white photos that tell the stories of children with disabilities playing and learning together.

Byars, Betsy. *The Summer of the Swans.* New York: Viking, 1970. A teen-aged girl gains insight into her priorities when her mentally challenged brother becomes lost.

Cairo, Shelley. *Our Brother Has Down's Syndrome.* New York: Annick, 1985. Children are introduced to Jai, a child with Down's Syndrome, and discover that the diffcrences between them and him are not so grcat.

Clifton, Lucille. *My Friend Jacob.* New York: Dutton, 1980. A young boy tells about Jacob, who though older, and mentally challenged, is his best friend.

Corcoran, Barbara. *A Dance to Still Music.* Ncw York: Atheneum, 1974. Fourteen-year-old Margaret runs in fear from the idea of attending a school for the deaf and meeting new people.

Garfield, James. *Follow My Leader.* New York: Viking Press, 1957. Eleven-year-old James finds himself visually impaired after an accident. This is a story of his acceptance of a disability and the various issues that surround this acceptance.

Girion, Barbara. *A Handful of Stars.* New York: Scribner, 1981. A senior high school girl named Julie must learn to live with epileptic seizures.

Howard, Ellen. *Circle of Giving.* New York: Atheneum, 1984. Margarite's world is changed when she meets Francie, a girl with cerebral palsy. Francie's mother finds the problem difficult to cope with and sees Francie as a burden.

Howe, James. *A Night Without Stars.* New York: Atheneum, 1983. Eleven-year-old Maria fears her heart surgery. "Monster Man," a person with horrible burn scars, helps her with her operation.

Kamisen, Janet. *What If You Couldn't . . . A Book About Special Needs.* New York: Scribner's, 1979. This book explains the causes and characteristics of other impairments as well as kinds of disabilities.

Keats, Ezra Jack. *Apt. 3.* New York: Macmillan, 1973. Two brothers search for a harmonica player in their apartment building. When they find him, they discover he is visually impaired, but has used his ears to learn a great deal about the world.

Little, Jean. *Mine for Keeps.* Boston: Little, Brown and Company, 1962. Sally, a young girl with cerebral palsy, comes home after being in a special needs school. This is a story about her struggle to adapt to her new environment.

Maclachlan, Patricia. *Through Grandpa's Eyes.* New York: Harper and Row. A young boy learns a different way of seeing the world from his visually impaired grandfather.

Morton, Jane. *Running Scared.* Wheaton, IL: Elsevier/Nelson Books, 1979. This is a work about a boy with a learning disability. The boy's inabilitiy to communicate well is frustrating for him. A counselor helps the child deal with these issues.

Pollock, Penny. *Keeping It Secret.* New York: Putnam, 1982. An eleven-year-old faces problems when she changes schools. She is hearing impaired; none of the other children in her classroom have impairments.

Powers, Mary Ellen. *Our Teacher's in a Wheelchair.* New York: Whitman, 1986. Text and photographs depict the activities of Brian Hanson, who is able to lead an active life as a nursery school teacher despite his partial paralysis.

Rabe, Bernice. *The Balancing Girl.* New York: Dutton. Margaret has developed the ability to balance all kinds of objects even though she uses a wheelchair. She balances magic markers and cans for her teachers. When she balances dominoes for the school fair, everyone sees her great skill.

Scott, Virgina. *Belonging.* Washington, DC: Gallaude University Press, 1986. Struck by meningitis at 15, a popular girl is physically devastated by her illness. She slowly gets her strength back, however, she loses her hearing.

Slote, Alfred. *Hang Tough, Paul Mather.* New York: Harper and Row, 1985. A young child struggles with his leukemia and hopes to continue to play sports.

Voigt, Cythia. *Izzy, Willy-Nilly.* New York: Atheneum, 1986. A young girl loses her legs in an accident. She must cope with her own emotions, her mother's denial, and her friends' discomfort.

REFERENCES

Bernstein, J. (1989). *Bibliotherapy: How books can help children cope.* In *Children's literature: Resource for the classroom* (Ed.) M. Rudman, 159-173. New York: Christopher Gordon Publishers, Inc.

Coleman, M., & Ganong, L. H. (1990). The use of juvenile fiction and self-help books with stepfamilies. *Journal of Counseling and Development,* 68, 327-331.

Ellis, A. (1993). The advantages and disadvantages of self-help therapy materials. *Professional Psychology, Research and Practice,* 24, 335-339.

Griffin, B. (1984). *Special needs bibliography: Current books for/about children and young adults.* DeWitt, NY: Griffin.

Hynes, A. M., & Wedl, L. C. (1990). Bibliotherapy: An interactive process in counseling older person. *Journal of Mental Health Counseling,* 21, 288-302.

McKinney, F. (1977). Exploration in bibliotherapy. *Personnel and Guidance Journal,* 56, 550-552.

Morris-Vann, A. M. (1979). *Once upon a time . . . A guide to the use of bibliotherapy.* Oak Park, MI: Aid-U Publishing Company.

Pardeck, J. T. (1998). *Using books in clinical social work practice: A guide to bibliotherapy.* New York: The Haworth Press, Inc.

Pardeck, J. T., & Musick, J. A. (2002). Recommended children's books on disabilities. *Journal of Social Work in Disability & Rehabilitation,* 1, 73-77.

Pardeck, J. A., & Pardeck, J. T. (1998). *Children in foster care and adoption: A guide to bibliotherapy.* Westport, CT: Greenwood Press.

Santrock, J. W., Minnett, A. M., & Campbell, B. D. (1994). *The authoritative guide to self-help books.* New York: The Guilford Press.

Shrodes, C. (1949). *Bibliotherapy: A theoretical and clinical study.* Doctoral Dissertation: University of California.

Starker, S. (1988). Psychologists and self-help books: Attitudes and prescriptive practices of clinicians. *American Journal of Psychotherapy,* 42, 448-455.

Webster's New Collegiate Dictionary. (1981). Springfield, MA: Merriam-Webster.

Zaccaria, J., & Moses, H. (1968). *Facilitating human development through reading: The use of bibliotherapy in teaching and counseling.* Champaign, IL: Stipes.

SECTION II
DISABILITY POLICY AND PROGRAMS
IN THE TWENTY-FIRST CENTURY

Reaching Out:
Evaluation of a Health Promotion Website
for Children with Disabilities
and Their Families

Virginia Rondero Hernandez
Katherine Selber
Mary Tijerina
Jennifer Mallow

Virginia Rondero Hernandez, PhD, is Assistant Professor, California State University, Fresno, Department of Social Work Education, Fresno, CA 93740-8019. Katherine Selber, PhD, is Associate Professor. Mary Tijerina, PhD, is Assistant Professor, and Jennifer Mallow, MSW, is a graduate of Texas State University, School of Social Work, San Marcos, TX 78666.

Address correspondence to: Katherine Selber at the above address.

The authors would like to acknowledge Hollie Reagan, MSW, Cathy Heyman, MA, Victor Gonzalez, MA and Sarah Maugans, MSW, for their work as Research Assistants on the project.

The research was supported in part by grants from the Texas Department of Health.

[Haworth co-indexing entry note]: "Reaching Out: Evaluation of a Health Promotion Website for Children with Disabilities and Their Families." Rondero Hernandez, Virginia et al. Co-published simultaneously in *Journal of Social Work in Disability & Rehabilitation* (The Haworth Social Work Practice Press, an imprint of The Haworth Press, Inc.) Vol. 4, No. 1/2, 2005, pp. 87-103; and: *Disability Issues for Social Workers and Human Services Professionals in the Twenty-First Century* (ed: John W. Murphy, and John T. Pardeck) The Haworth Social Work Practice Press, an imprint of The Haworth Press, Inc., 2005, pp. 87-103. Single or multiple copies of this article are available for a fee from The Haworth Document Delivery Service [1-800-HAWORTH, 9:00 a.m. - 5:00 p.m. (EST). E-mail address: docdelivery@haworthpress.com].

87

SUMMARY. This article describes how a state health authority capitalized on the increased popularity of the Internet among consumers by launching a website devoted to improving communication among persons interested in children with disabilities and their families. The health authority collaborated with a local school of social work to redesign the website using the family-centered paradigm and evaluate its effectiveness. A sample of 51 respondents participated in the web-based survey. The article describes the process and methods of evaluation as well as the results of the survey to enhance feedback for the website's further development. Lessons learned for the design, development, and marketing of future websites are also covered. *[Article copies available for a fee from The Haworth Document Delivery Service: 1-800-HAWORTH. E-mail address: <docdelivery@haworthpress.com> Website: <http://www.HaworthPress.com> © 2005 by The Haworth Press, Inc. All rights reserved.]*

KEYWORDS. Disability, website, web-based survey, family-centered services

As the Internet continues to grow and revolutionize the process of disseminating and gathering information, an increasing number of consumers as well as health and human service organizations are turning to it as a tool for a variety of purposes (Princeton Survey Research Associates, 2001). According to the United States Census Bureau (2001), 54 million households, or 51 percent, had one or more computers and 42 percent had access to the Internet at home as of August 2000. Many of these people turn to the Internet before consulting a health professional. According to the Pew Internet Project (2000), two-thirds of all Americans expect to find reliable health care information online with an estimated 73 million Americans having gone online in search of health information. The Internet offers the advantage for consumers to gather information at their own speed, from their own home or work at minimal expense.

In addition, in a survey of human service providers there was strong support for the use of information technology in the helping professions (Hughes, Joo, Zentall, & Ulishney, 1999). Many health and human service organizations use the Internet to accomplish a variety of mission-based functions including health promotion activities and community education (Finn, 2000; Hughes et al., 1999; Schoech, 2002). These organizations are discovering that promoting public awareness of social and health topics using the Internet serves to enhance their effectiveness in the community by educating consumers in a cost effective and current manner. Social workers, educators, health professionals, and even caretakers themselves have acknowledged the importance of the Internet for seeking information, services, and monitoring accountability of service systems.

Such functions as seeking information and services are particularly important in the area of disability practice where families must often deal with multiple agencies and systems for obtaining needed services (Tijerina, Selber, & Rondero Hernandez, 2003). For example, it is common for families of children with disabilities to require services from a myriad number of systems including health, rehabilitation, school, legal, and mental health systems of care. This involvement with multiple service systems often requires consumers to bridge gaps in service or distinguish the overlapping of services in order to gain access to the services they desire for their family member. This type of activity underscores the importance of accessing information in ways that recognize the needs of families with children with disabilities as well as other stakeholders such as professionals who serve this population.

This article describes how a state health authority capitalized on the increased popularity of the Internet among consumers by launching a website devoted to improving communication among persons interested in children with disabilities and their families. The original primary focus of the website was to educate communities about conditions among individuals with disabilities and how to prevent them from occurring. After establishing that the original site needed improvement, the health authority collaborated with a university's school of social work to develop a new website and evaluate its effectiveness. The article describes the process and methods of evaluation as well as the results of a pilot study to enhance feedback for the website's development. Lessons learned for the design, development, and marketing of future websites will also be covered. In addition, policy and practice implications will be offered.

ENHANCING ACCESS
WITHIN A FAMILY-CENTERED FOCUS

The website evaluation formed part of a larger project to assist the state health authority with a federally funded capacity-building project to enhance state services for families with children with disabilities. The focus of the overall project was to strengthen the capability of existing services for centering services around the needs of families first and foremost. In order to develop a more effective website, its developers utilized the literature of family-centered care to conceptualize and incorporate consumer-friendly features.

Current literature indicates that quality of life may be enhanced by interventions that engage the family and are sensitive to their needs. Family-centered care is a concept that represents a consumer-oriented model of care that treats an individual with special needs and their family with respect and dignity (Johnson, 1999, 2000). Family-centered care appears as a concept found in the literature of family-centered planning (FCP), and advocates for the development of service delivery systems that are responsive to family needs (Patterson, Garwick, Bennett, & Blum, 1997). According to this model, families are viewed as the experts on their child and are expected to participate equally with care providers regarding their children's needs and treatment (Simeonsson, Edmondson, Smith, Sarnahan, & Bucy, 1995; D'Antuono, 1998). One of the core values of this model is the importance of respecting the family's values, environment, culture, resources, needs, and strengths (D'Antuono, 1998), and viewing these characteristics as assets for patient care and treatment plans (Trivette, Dunst, & Hamby, 1996; Allen & Petr, 1998; Ahmann & Johnson, 2000). In addition, family-centered models view the family as the primary context for promoting health, and place the family at the center of service design and delivery activities (Dunst, Illback, & Cobb, 1997).

Although there are dissenting opinions about the value and implementation of family-centered care (Dunst, Johanson, Trivette, & Hamby, 1991; Powell, 1996), research on family-centered models of care has gained momentum in a variety of areas over the last decade, including work with families of children with chronic illness, developmental disabilities, early childhood intervention programs, rehabilitation programs, and mental health systems of care (Patterson, Garwick, Bennett, & Blum, 1997; Bailey, McWilliam, Darkes, Hebbler, Simeonsson, Spiker, & Wagner, 1998). Discussion about family-centered care is linked with discussions about improving the quality of life for people with disabilities (Gibson, 1995; King, Rosenbaum, & King, 1997). Concepts and recommendations from this literature base were used to enhance the promotion of health authority services, including the website, to families with children with disabilities across the state.

OVERALL WEBSITE DESIGN

The state health authority's original website was very basic in both its content and design. Overall, the site provided few links and there was no clear pattern of how the user was to navigate through the information they were viewing. Therefore, it was difficult for users to retrace their steps and get back to the needed information. Anecdotal feedback from users of the website indicated that the site segregated information between parents and professionals. Visitors did not view the content found on the site as information the general population of families could use, and they commented that the site was inclined to use professional language rather than language of a general consumer. This pointed to the fact that consumers did not find the site either consumer-friendly or family-oriented. As a result of this feedback, the health authority staff and the university team decided the website needed to follow the overall project's emphasis and be redesigned to incorporate a more family-centered approach. It was determined that the site needed improvements to both its design as well as its content. The purpose of redesigning the website then was twofold. Conceptually, the redesign needed to follow a more family-centered focus. In terms of practice, the redesign needed to make it more visually appealing, easier to navigate, and more informative.

WEBSITE REDESIGN PROCESS

To gather ideas for creating the new site, other websites in the fields of disabilities and rehabilitation were examined for ideas on design, color schemes, and layout. This step yielded concrete ideas for the layout and overall look of the site. The first step in restructuring the website was to re-categorize each page on the site by topics and then rename the corresponding pages. All content found on the site was consolidated and duplicate information deleted.

The university team also reviewed the website for People First language. A variety of health and human services professionals as well as staff working in the field of disability reviewed the content for People First language. As part of this process, the website was also reviewed by the project's Advisory Board members including families with children with disabilities and advocates within the disability field.

To further improve the website for people with disabilities, the university team went through the process of becoming "Bobby-Approved."

Bobby is a web accessibility software tool designed to identify and repair barriers to accessibility. Bobby tests Web pages using the guidelines established by the World Wide Web Consortium's (W3C) Web Access Initiative, as well as U.S. Section 508 guidelines from the Architectural and Transportation Barriers Compliance Board, Web Accessibility Guidelines (World Wide Web Consortium, 2004).

People with disabilities can experience difficulty using the Web due to a combination of barriers in the information on Web pages and barriers in the browsers, multimedia players, or assistive technologies such as screen readers or voice recognition. The guidelines provide specific help to Web page developers in order to prevent people with disabilities from having problems accessing information in a thorough and easy manner. Such issues as images without texts, un-described video, or sites with poor color contrast can create challenges for people with a variety of physical, visual, hearing, and cognitive disabilities (World Wide Web Consortium, 2004).

Once the redesigned site was completed it was given to a contractor to be implemented. The resulting website featured more concise content, was less cumbersome to navigate, offered less redundant information, and was faster to download. The new website was titled "On the Right Track: Improving Health for People with Special Needs" (ORT).

WEBSITE PROMOTION

In order to market the new website and build an audience, information was disseminated regarding its redesign. A brochure was developed explaining the purpose of the new website, identifying the developmental disabilities the site featured, and explaining the benefits of its use. The brochure was used to promote the website at a variety of conferences, meetings, health promotion community activities, and as a routine part of communicating with stakeholders within the larger overall project. The second step was the development of a PowerPoint slide show presentation on the website which covered the primary features of the website such as its goals, the way the information was organized, and the type of information covered. This presentation was shared at three statewide professional conferences in order to encourage attendees to visit the site when they returned to their agency. In addition the slide show was also used at meetings and focus groups for other goals of the overall project.

METHOD

Four months after restructuring the website, the university team conducted an evaluation of the website's design, content, and usefulness. Several questions guided the survey. First, does the web design allow users to access information easily? Is the content of the information provided useful to its users? Is the website visually appealing?

The field of web-based surveys is still relatively new (Epstein & Klinkenberg, 2002; Petit, 1999; Sorensen, 2001). Current literature on the use of this methodology often describes the pros and cons of such surveys. The problems associated with the methodology include such issues as sampling problems, lack of control over the experimental environment, and data collection problems. The benefits identified include access to difficult to reach populations, ease of data collection, and greater disclosure from respondents due to a lack of face-to-face contact (Epstein & Klinkenberg, 2002; Schultz, Fawcett, Francisco, Wolff, Berkowitz, & Nagy, 2000).

The website redesign and evaluation formed part of an overall project to examine various stakeholder perceptions of existing services and gaps and to research the feasibility of moving to a more family-centered system design. Hence, it was decided that the use of a web-based survey would be a consistent methodology. Since the review of a website should be done electronically, not in a paper and pencil manner, it seemed logical that its evaluation would likewise be electronically driven. In addition, there were administrative issues of both time and resources that supported the argument for an electronic evaluation. A web-based survey offered the advantage of collecting survey data quickly and inexpensively. Current literature indicates that web-based surveys are the ideal universal medium for collecting and disseminating large amounts of information because they can be accessed through various operating system platforms and across geographic distances (Flowers, Bray, & Algozzine, 1999; Schoech, 2002). Since the website development and evaluation was part of a statewide project, reaching a wider audience outside of the local area was of paramount importance. The state health agency endorsed this innovative application.

Instrumentation

After conducting a review of the literature, and a broad Internet based research of surveys available on the Internet, the university team decided to customize a survey to evaluate the new website. The survey was modeled after the survey the Centers for Disease Control and Prevention used to evaluate its website in the spring of 2001 (CDC, 2001). The ORT survey was comprised of 31 nominal, categorical, and open-ended questions. The survey instrument used was piloted for the first time on this evaluation effort, thus, no data on reliability and validity were available.

To assist in the design of the evaluation survey and facilitate data collection and analysis efforts, the team researched commercial software to support the web-based survey. Numerous web-based surveys that were designed and published using a variety of software were reviewed. Survey Solutions by the Pursues Development Corporation was chosen primarily due to the positive testimonials and recommendation from consumers and researchers who had used the software to solicit customer feedback, or evaluate customer satisfaction and other consumer- related topics. The features found most appealing were the software's ease of use, availability of technical assistance, and low cost. The consumer-oriented design of the software's capability was also of critical importance given the family-centered paradigm used in the overall project.

Participants

Snowball and convenience sampling strategies were utilized to recruit potential participants for this study in one of two ways. The first set of participants was identified through existing listservs targeted at audiences interested in disabilities, special health care needs of children, and advocacy for persons with disabilities. This resulted in a total of six listservs and all their members received an invitation to participate in the survey. Listserv members were primarily caregivers of one or more children with developmental disabilities, professionals, and/or family members interested in issues related to developmental disabilities. The second set of invitations went to individuals identified by the state health authority staff and the university team. These individuals included university faculty and students, state-level employees, advocacy groups, and persons with developmental disabilities and their family members. Based on listserv sizes and an audit of individual emails reported, it is estimated that approximately 1,500 listserv members and other individuals received an invitation to participate in the web-based survey. These sampling techniques, although appropriate for a pilot survey, have limitations in terms of representativeness and generalizability. Thus, the results of the survey can only be viewed as exploratory in nature and may not be useful in other website evaluation efforts (Rubin & Babbie, 2001).

Procedure

Notice of the survey was announced on the new website, the university's web page, and by electronic invitation to listserv members and individuals identified by the state health authority and the university team. The electronic invitation provided an overview of the overall project, stated the purpose of the survey, and encouraged potential subjects to visit and evaluate the website. The electronic invitation was disseminated twice, in one week intervals. The first invitation went to 495 email addresses and six listservs. Out of the initial 495 individual emails, 94 (19%) were sent back stating that the recipients' email addresses were not current. The second invitation was sent the following week and went to 401 individuals. None from the second invitation were returned, indicating successful contact with the recipient.

Through the duration of the survey an electronic invitation was posted on the websites of both the state health authority and the university research team. The electronic invitation explained the purpose of the survey, informed the participant that participation was voluntary, and guaranteed anonymity. The University's Institutional Review Board (IRB) approval was also mentioned in the invitation to participate and on the website. Consent to participate was implied by the subject's completion of the survey, although subjects were given the option to initiate or discontinue the survey after reading the purpose of the study. A link to the survey was located at the end of the invitation to attract the attention of persons who found the site through search engines. The survey was posted for seven weeks.

RESULTS

Participants

The survey yielded a total of 51 participants or a total rate of return of about 13% (N = 401). This rate of return represents a considerable limitation of the study. Although not uncommon in web-based survey efforts, the return rate limits generalizability of the results (Epstein & Klinkenberg, 2002; Rubin & Babbie, 2001). The demographics of the sample are presented in Table 1. Most of the participants were female

TABLE 1. Demographics of Participants

Characteristics	Percent
Gender	
Male	22.9
Female	70.8
Declined to answer	6.3
Location	
In state	84.3
Out of state	7.8
Declined to answer	7.8
Internet Usage	
Daily basis	92.2
Weekly basis	7.8
Role of Participant	
Family member of person with disability	26.5
Person with a disability	2
Physician	2
Health care provider	38.8
Educator	4.1
Public agency administrative staff	12.2
Advocate for people with disabilities	28.6
Other	26.5

(70.8%), lived in-state (84.3%), and were daily users of the Internet (92.2%). For the most part, the participants identified themselves as health care providers (38.8%), advocates for people with disabilities (26.5%), family members of a person with a disability (26.5%), and administrative staff of public agencies (12.2%).

Family-Centered Content

Participants were asked to answer "yes," "no," or "I am not familiar with family-centered planning" to whether or not they were familiar with the concept of "family-centered planning" prior to viewing the ORT website. Out of the 51 participants, 78.4% participants answered "yes," 15.7% said "no" and 5.9% said they were "still not familiar with family-centered planning." Participants were also asked whether or not the family centered concept is important to individuals who work with and care for children with special health care needs. Ninety-eight percent (n = 50) of the participants thought family-centered planning was important to individuals who work with and care for children with disabilities. Another 2% answered that they were "not sure" if it was important.

Evaluation of the Website

When subjects were asked if the site was easy to navigate, 94.1% (n = 48) said yes, while only 5.9% (n = 3) answered no. Seventy-eight percent (n = 39) of the participants stated that they found the amount of information on the site to be just about right; 14% (n = 7) found it to be overwhelming; and 8% (n = 4) found that there was not enough. Participants were provided a Likert scale ranging from "excellent" to "poor" to rate the overall case of reading of the ORT website (i.e., fonts, background, page arrangement): 92.2% of the participants answered "excellent" or "very good"; 3.9% said "average"; and 3.9% marked "fair."

Participants were asked to provide an overall ranking for the website using a Likert scale containing the following categories: "excellent"; "very good"; "satisfactory"; "below average"; or "not good." Of the 51 respondents, 29.4% said it was "excellent"; 54.9% said "very good"; 9.8% said "satisfactory," 3.9% said "below average," and 2% said "not good."

DISCUSSION

The online survey represented a formal effort to assess and evaluate the approach, design, content, and usefulness of the website among consumer groups. The number of individuals who responded to the survey represents only a small percentage of those contacted, less than a 4% return rate; thus, little can be generalized from the study to other similar web-based efforts. The low response rate was likely due to the limited amount of time the university team was able to post the website before the evaluation was conducted. The website redesign and the evaluation invitations were only viewed for a little less than two months before data collection was ended. The lack of a lengthier timeline was primarily the result of delays in securing the required IRB approval, as well as other time demands placed on the overall project as it neared completion. These delays and time demands resulted in less time to collect responses about the website than had previously been planned. This short timeline is not comparable to other similar web-based data collection efforts that often allow as long as eight months for web-based data collection efforts to proceed (Epstein & Klinkenburg, 2002).

Surprisingly, 80.4% (n = 41) of the participants were viewing the website for the first time. This seemed to indicate that the electronic invitation for the survey ultimately served two purposes. First, the invitation solicited consumer and provider feedback. Second, it provided publicity of the website's existence to approximately 1,500 individuals and listserv members. The high percentage of first time users is important to note. This indicates that the site needed to be more widely publicized in order to maximize its full potential of making people aware of the importance of information on disability and family-centered approaches to service delivery.

Participants were also asked to select what Internet browser they used when they were online. Out of the five choices they were given the two most common browsers were Internet Explorer (72.5%) and Netscape (21.6%). It is important that web developers are sensitive to what browsers their visitors are using because there are variations in how browsers interpret Hyper-Text Markup Language (HTML). Different browsers may display the websites differently. For example, the site's text may look like the developer intends in Internet Explorer, but in Netscape all the text may appear underlined.

The survey results showed that people who viewed the new site found it to be easy to navigate, easy to read and the amount of information was helpful and not burdensome. The university team and the health authority staff concluded that the redesign of the website was successful in reaching the goals of creating a website that was informative and consumer friendly.

IMPLICATIONS AND LESSONS LEARNED

The university team identified many lessons learned after building, maintaining, and evaluating the website during the year-and-a-half of work on the overall project. The experiences included the review of approximately 2,000 different websites, as well as the formal feedback obtained from the survey participants, and informal discussions with professionals, family members, and other website masters about how to develop, maintain and evaluate a website for the field of disability services. The lessons learned include those concerning website maintenance, additions of databases/links, usefulness of e-mail newsletters, and the importance of obtaining on-going feedback from website users.

The first step in maintaining a website is to have the capability of running the site through an application to check for current links. This process checks the site for internal and external broken links and then fixes or replaces them. This requires additional time and research. The second step in maintaining the website is to search the Internet, on a regular basis, for new links to keep the website current. As part of this activity, it became important to also monitor several listservs within the disability field. These electronic communities of parents and caregivers as well as professionals have been found to be a useful resource in identifying what parents and caregivers of children with disabilities want and need. This activity helps to maintain a family-centered focus.

The importance of maintaining websites on a regular basis cannot be underestimated. The literature on website marketing speaks to the necessity of actively maintaining the website as the first and most important step in any thorough marketing plan (Au & Tipton, 2000). The goal of actively maintaining the website is, of course, both to prevent losing frequent visitors due to the perception that the site is outdated and to help attract new visitors by having reliable and timely information. While researching approximately 2,000 websites, it became apparent that the websites that receive high volumes of traffic appear to be those sites that are maintained and updated on a regular basis. In addition, these websites also appear to be networked with other sites that share common areas of interest. This means considerable time must be allocated to requesting linkages with other websites as a proactive way of marketing the site.

Current research states that many of the individuals in your target audience visit your website because of something they have read, not because they are looking for your site via a search engine (Cravens, 2000). With this in mind, it is recommended that staff find additional ways of increasing website traffic such as the distribution of a monthly electronic newsletter sent via email as one way to publicize the site. New information from a project can be shared in the newsletter as well as providing a method of discussing new features of the website.

Finally, staff should provide a way to obtain continuous feedback regarding the website. As an on-line tool for consumers, it is important that the information provided on the website reflect the needs of the consumers and that the site be easy to read and navigate. Therefore, it is recommended that a brief survey be added as a permanent feature to the site. Some suggested questions are: What Internet browser do you use when viewing this website? How did you find out about the website? How often do you visit the site? Overall, did you find the website easy to read? Overall, did you find the site easy to navigate? Please share your suggestions for improving this website or any additional comments you might have. The purpose of the brief, on-going survey would be to provide quality assurance on the website and ensure that the website is meeting consumers' needs.

A final lesson learned included the tendency to underestimate the time and technical expertise needed to design, maintain, and evaluate a website. This effort consumed the majority of one full-time staff person. A lack of technical expertise commonly exists in the information technology (IT) area within human service organizations (Princeton Survey Research Associates, 2001). This can lead to a significant underestimation of the time and effort needed to adequately perform this role and jeopardize the success and effectiveness of a website. In addition, it is very helpful to have experience in the field of disability practice in addition to IT skills. Having both sets of knowledge and skills makes it easier to select relevant content for the website and make the website pertinent to the needs of its users.

This research experience also points to the need to enhance curriculum in schools of social work within the areas of information technology, marketing, and health promotion for persons with disabilities. Literature already suggests that social work lags behind other helping professions in terms of inclusion of information on disabilities (Pardeck, 2001). These topics are not covered in-depth or regularly across social work programs. Although IT is being used with increasing frequency in social work programs for classroom support and distance education, more emphasis on in-depth skill development in this area is important for the employment of future social work graduates. If changes in practice regarding the improvement of IT use within the health and human services field are to be gained, such changes must parallel changes in both undergraduate and graduate social work curricula.

The study results also point to policy and practice implications. In terms of policy, the study points to the need to strengthen efforts at providing services in a family-centered framework. Too often, agency policy-makers design their services without sufficient input from families. The result can be limited access to services and decreased usefulness to families, especially in the field of disability services where families often are using services from many systems of care (Tijerina, Selber, & Rondero Hernandez, 2004). Seeking input from families around policies, service design and implementation issues, and evaluation is essential.

In terms of practice, the usefulness of web-based services cannot be over emphasized. This requires a commitment from managers of human service providers to think through the implications of their websites for people seeking services and for other professionals accessing information to make appropriate referrals. The field of health and human services will continue to rely on web-based efforts for a range of service provision as budgets are reprioritized in the wake of September 11, 2001. This implies that managers must also understand the need to have staff trained in technology and human services so that websites can be designed combining both sets of skills.

In addition, there are implications for the use of technology in the field of disabilities services as well as other health and human services. The Internet is a powerful tool for health promotion due to its multimedia capacity and the proliferation of access. Health and human service organizations, especially within the field of disability practice, still lag behind other sectors in Internet and IT utilization (Schoech, 2002). Although this gap appears to be narrowing, the question of how to not only use these tools but how best to use them for such efforts as website development and collecting data from consumers in different locations with diverse interests and needs remains an important topic for future research. Problems associated with web-based research such as sampling error and bias, suggests caution in embracing the tool without careful consideration of future study limitations (Gonzalez, 2002). However, social work educators as well as other health and human service professionals must begin to teach these tools both in terms of a knowledge base and skills. Only with such academic-based efforts will the issues associated with these methods and tools be addressed.

REFERENCES

Ahmann, E., & Johnson, B. (2000, January). Family-centered care: Facing the new millennium [Interview]. *Pediatric Nursing* [Online] 26(1). Available: http://newfirst search.oclc.org (Accessed 16, March 2001).

Allen, R. I., & Petr, C. G. (1998). Rethinking family-centered practice. *American Journal of Orthopsychiatry, 68*(1), 4-15.

Au, K., & Tipton, R. (2000, November 3). Internet marketing for non-profit organizations. *Owl'sRoost* [Online] Available: http://www-rci.rutgers.edu/~au/workshop/imarket.htm#A (Accessed 19, July 2001).

Bailey, D. B., McWilliam, R. A., Darkes, L. A., Hebbler, K., Simeonsson, R. J., Spiker, D., & Wagner, M. (1998, Spring). Family outcomes in early intervention: A framework for program evaluation and efficacy research. *Exceptional Children, 64*(3), 313-328.

Centers for Disease Control and Prevention (2001). Website Evaluation Instrument. [Online] Available: *http://outside.cdc.gov:8091/BASIS/survey/survey/survey/upf* (Accessed April, 2001).

Cravens, J. (2000, August 7). Marketing your web site both offline and online. *Coyote Communication* [Online] Available: http://www.coyotecom.com/webdevo/webmrkt.html (Accessed 19, July 2001).

D'Antuono, R. (1998). Good business. *Academic Clinical Practice* [Online] *11*(4). Available: http://www.aamc.org (Accessed 01, January 2001).

Dunst, C. J., Illback, R. J., & Cobb, C. T. (1997). Conceptual and empirical foundations of family-centered practice: Opportunities for psychological practice. R. J. Illback, & C. T. Cobb (Eds.) (pp. 75-91). Washington, DC: American Psychological Association.

Dunst, C. J., Johanson, C., Trivette, C. M., & Hamby, D. (1991, October/November). Family-oriented early intervention policies and practices: Family-centered or not? *Exceptional Children, 58*(2), 115-126.

Epstein, J., & Klinkenberg, W. (2002). Collecting data via the Internet: The development and deployment of a web-based survey. *Journal of Technology in Human Services, 19*, 33-47.

Finn, J. (2000). A survey of domestic violence organizations on the world wide web. *Journal of Human Service Technology, 17*, 83-102.

Flowers, C. P., Bray, M., & Algozzine, R. F. (1999). Accessibility of special education program home pages. *Journal of Special Education Technology* [Online] *14*(2). Available: http://relayweb.hwwilsonweb.com (Accessed 19, February 2001).

Gibson, C. H. (1995). The process of empowerment in mothers of chronically ill children. *Journal of Advanced Nursing, 21*, 1201-1210.

Gonzalez, J. E. (2002). Present day use of the Internet for survey-based research. *Journal of Technology in Human Services, 19*, 19-31.

Hughes, R., Joo, E., Zentall, S., & Ulishney, K. (1999). Access and use of information technology by human service providers. *Journal of Technology in Human Services, 16*, 1-16.

Johnson, B. (2000). Family-centered care: Four decades of progress. *The Journal of Collaborative Family Healthcare, 18*, 137-147.

Johnson, B. H. (1999, March). Family Focus. *Trustee, 52*(3), 12-15.

King, G. A., Rosenbaum, P. L., & King, S. M. (1997). Evaluating family-centered service using a measure of parents' perceptions. *Child: Care, Health, and Development, 23*(1), 47-62.

Pardeck, J. (2001). Editorial: A critical analysis of the social work literature on disabilities. *Journal of Social Work in Disability & Rehabilitation, 1*, 1, 1-3.

Patterson, J. M., Garwick, A. W., Bennett, F. C., & Blum, R. (1997, December). Social support in families of children with chronic conditions: Supportive and nonsupportive behaviors. *Journal of Developmental and Behavioral Pediatrics, 18*(6), 383-391.

Pettit, F. (1999). Exploring the use of the World Wide Web as a psychology data collection tool. *Computers in Human Behavior, 15,* 67-71.

Pew Foundation (2000). The online health care revolution: How the web helps Americans take better care of themselves. Retrieved April 30, 2003 from the Pew Internet and American Life Project web site *http://www.pewinternet.org/reports/toc.asp?Report=26*

Powell, J. Y. (1996, September). A schema for family-centered practice. *Families in Society: The Journal of Contemporary Human Services,* pp. 446-448.

Princeton Survey Research Associates (2001). *Wired, Willing and Ready: NonProfit Human Service Organizations' Adoption of Information Technology.* Available on-line at: *http://www.independentsector.org/media/WiredWillingReadyPR.html* (Retrieved September 1, 2003).

Rubin, Allen, & Babbie, Earl (2001). *Research Methods for Social Work.* Belmont, CA: Wadsworth/Thomas Learning.

Schoech, D. (2002). Technology challenges facing social work. *Electronic Journal of Social Work, 1,* 1. Available on-line at *http://www.e/sw.net.*

Schultz, J., Fawcett, S., Francisco, V., Wolff, T., Berkowitz, B., & Nagy, G. (2000). The community tool box: Using the Internet to support the work of community health and development. *Journal of Technology in Human Services, 17,* 193-215.

Simeonsson, R. J., Bailey, D., Smith, T., & Buysse, V. (1995, December). Young children with disabilities: Functional assessment by teachers. *Journal of Developmental & Physical Disabilities, 7*(4), 267-284.

Sorensen, A. (2001). Promoting public health through electronic media: A challenge for schools of public health. *Journal of Public Health, 91,* 1182-1185.

Tijerina, M., Selber, K., and Rondero Hernandez, V. (2004). Perceptions of the Texas genetics services system and genetic information needs of health care providers: A web-based survey. *Texas Journal of Rural Health, 21*(4), 35-43.

Trivette, C. M., Dunst, C. J., & Hamby, D. W. (1996). Factors associated with perceived control appraisals in a family-centered early intervention program. *Journal of Early Intervention, 20*(2), 165-170.

U.S. Census Bureau (2001). Home computers and Internet use in the United States. Retrieved April 30, 2003 from the US Census web site: *http://www.census.gov/prod/2001pubs/p23-207.pdf*

World Wide Web Consortium (2004). Accessibility Guidelines. Retrieved January 13, 2004 from the World Wide Web Consortium website *http://www.w3.org/WAI/Resources/#in*

Rural and Urban Differences Among Mental Health Consumers in One Midwestern State: Implications for Policy, Practice, and Research

John Q. Hodges

Martha Markward

Dong Pil Yoon

Carol J. Evans

John Q. Hodges, PhD, is Assistant Professor, University of Missouri, Columbia, School of Social Work, 721 Clark Hall, Columbia, MO 65211. Martha Markward, PhD, is Associate Professor, University of Missouri, Columbia, School of Social Work, 718 Clark Hall, Columbia, MO 65211. Dong Pil Yoon, PhD, is Assistant Professor, University of Missouri, Columbia, School of Social Work, 701 Clark Hall, Columbia, MO 65211. Carol J. Evans, PhD, is Director, Child and Family Mental Health Services Research Division, Missouri Institute of Mental Health, 5400 Arsenal Street, Saint Louis, MO 63139.

The authors wish to thank Cynthia Keele, Executive Director, Missouri National Alliance for the Mentally Ill, for all her work and support on this project.

This research was financially supported by the National Alliance for the Mentally Ill of Missouri and the University of Missouri, Columbia.

[Haworth co-indexing entry note]: "Rural and Urban Differences Among Mental Health Consumers in One Midwestern State: Implications for Policy, Practice, and Research." Hodges, John Q. et al. Co-published simultaneously in *Journal of Social Work in Disability & Rehabilitation* (The Haworth Social Work Practice Press, an imprint of The Haworth Press, Inc.) Vol. 4, No. 1/2, 2005, pp. 105-120; and: *Disability Issues for Social Workers and Human Services Professionals in the Twenty-First Century* (ed: John W. Murphy, and John T. Pardeck) The Haworth Social Work Practice Press, an imprint of The Haworth Press, Inc., 2005, pp. 105-120. Single or multiple copies of this article are available for a fee from The Haworth Document Delivery Service [1-800-HAWORTH, 9:00 a.m. - 5:00 p.m. (EST). E-mail address: docdelivery@haworthpress.com].

SUMMARY. This study examines differences in rural and urban mental health service utilization and service satisfaction. A cross-sectional survey design was used to gather information from a sample of 311 mental health consumers regarding their use of services relative to accessibility, availability, affordability, and acceptability. Data were collected from respondents individually or in small groups in various locations in one Midwestern state. Study findings showed that rural consumers are aware of fewer services, use fewer services, and are less satisfied with services than are urban consumers. Implications for rural mental health policy, practice, and future research are discussed. *[Article copies available for a fee from The Haworth Document Delivery Service: 1-800-HAWORTH. E-mail address: <docdelivery@haworthpress.com> Website: <http://www.HaworthPress. com> © 2005 by The Haworth Press, Inc. All rights reserved.]*

KEYWORDS. Rural, urban, mental health, service utilization, service satisfaction, consumer

Approximately 60 million Americans (or slightly less than one-fourth of the U.S. population) live in rural areas; these rural citizens have similar rates of mental illness and substance abuse disorders as their urban counterparts, as well as similar need for services (Wagenfeld & Murray et al., 1994; Mohatt, 1997; National Institute of Mental Health, 2000). However, significant differences have been found in availability of care, access to care (financial and otherwise), and quality of care for rural residents (NIMH, 2000). These service utilization differences are often framed in terms of accessibility, availability, affordability, and acceptability (Stefl & Prosperi, 1985; Bushy, 1997).

Given that the Americans With Disabilities Act (ADA) of 1990 includes mental illness among covered disabilities, these rural/urban difficulties in service usage become even more salient. Psychiatric rehabilitation programs and advocates for those with mental illnesses are calling for more equitable access to services under the ADA (Granger & Gill, 2000). All agencies working with mentally ill clients, whether public or private, urban or rural, have an obligation to ensure their services are accessible under the ADA (Rinere & Morris, 1997). In this study, we examined differences between urban and rural mental health consumers in these four areas (accessibility, availability, affordability, and acceptability) using consumer input in the creation and administration of the research instrument, as well as the use of a service satisfaction scale with good psychometric properties.

BACKGROUND/RATIONALE

Service accessibility, availability, affordability, and acceptability present problems for persons seeking mental health services in rural areas. For example, availability of and access to services are often problems in rural areas for a variety of reasons (NIMH, 2000). Affordability is another problem that is especially salient in rural areas where many persons lack financial resources to access treatment. Finally, there is often little acceptability of mental health as a legitimate condition in many rural areas, and as a result, persons who seek help for mental health problems are often stigmatized.

Availability/Accessibility. A number of factors are associated with the availability of and access to mental health services in rural areas. Consumers are likely to lack information on what services are available and where to go for services. Further, when services are available, they frequently require the consumer to travel great distances to access those services. In many cases, rural mental health services also lack the breadth of service type seen in urban areas. Crisis services and peer support groups are particularly scarce in rural areas (Maine Rural Health Research Center, 1999a,b).

Lower population density and fewer numbers of consumers dictate that mental health is seldom a priority in rural budgets. Consequently, rural residents may rely upon informal helping networks such as family, friends, or religious affiliations to assist with problems. Further, there is often an insufficient infrastructure in rural areas, which also contributes to low numbers of professional mental health providers (Bushy, 1997; MRHRC, 1999a,b; NIMH, 2000). For example, over 60% of rural areas have been designated as "Federal Mental Health Professional Shortage Areas" (Mohatt, 1997). This lack of professional mental health providers in rural areas cuts across disciplines, including psychology, psychiatry, and social work (Mohatt & Kirwan, 1995).

When mental health services are sought in rural areas, general medical practitioners frequently deliver them, with minimal or no training in treating mental disorders. Access to self-help services is often limited, consumer and family input is commonly devalued, and quality of mental health care may not match that found in urban areas (Schurman, Kramer, & Mitchell, 1985; MRHRC, 1999b). Many mental health professionals in rural areas are trained as specialists, rather than generalists who are able to take on a variety of necessary roles such as therapist, case manager, community educator, and grant writer (Bushy, 1997).

The concept of "least restrictive care" is often unavailable or unfeasible for rural consumers. In general, only 79.5 percent of rural counties have mental health services (Hartley, Bird, & Dempsey, 1999). The range of services in rural areas is narrower than that in urban areas. When crisis services are unavailable, a rural consumer is more likely to be hospitalized than an urban consumer who has access to preventative services such as crisis lines, peer support, and psychiatric emergency services (MHRHC, 1999b). Hospitalization, however, may not exist in close proximity to a consumer's home. Many rural areas lack access to inpatient psychiatric care altogether, forcing consumers to be hospitalized many miles from their home communities (Mohatt, 1997). To illustrate, while 95% of urban counties have inpatient psychiatric services, only 13% of rural counties have these services (Wagenfeld, Goldsmith, Stiles, & Manderscheid, 1988). When hospitalization is available in rural areas, inpatient care is often of lower quality than that found in urban areas (NIMH, 2000).

Affordability. Financial barriers to treatment are also prevalent in rural areas (NIMH, 2000). While rural consumers may qualify for financial benefits such as Medicaid, Medicare, and Social Security, they are less likely to have case managers, case aides, or peer-advocacy organizations to help them negotiate the bureaucratic challenges to obtaining these benefits. For example, the results in one study found that only 25% of people in rural areas qualified for Medicaid (compared to 43% in urban areas), despite very high rates of poverty in rural areas. Further, those in rural areas often had less comprehensive insurance plans, which typically did not cover the cost of mental health care (MRHRC, 1999a; NIMH, 2000); in addition, they were more likely to have no insurance when compared to urban residents (Mohatt, 1997). Even when rural residents have comparable insurance, they use fewer services than do urban residents (when controlling for the effects of disease presence and severity). For example, rural Medicaid recipients with depression use fewer services than urban beneficiaries. This finding has been linked to the afore-mentioned deficit of mental health professionals in rural areas (Maine Rural Health Research Center, 1997).

Acceptability. While stigma is a problem for most mental health consumers in the United States, rural consumers face unique issues in this regard. Although there is great diversity among rural communities (Bushy, 1997; National Rural Health Association, 1999), many retain cultural and societal values that stigmatize not only mental illness itself, but also the act of seeking help for the illness (Hoyt, Conger, Valde, & Weihs, 1997; NIMH, 2000). This is often attributed to rural values of self-reliance and/or reliance upon family rather than "outsiders" (Bushy, 1997). When help is sought, it is often sought from general medical practitioners, due to a lack of mental health providers and because it is more acceptable in many rural cultures to seek treatment for physical ailments rather than mental ones (NHRA, 1999).

In addition to cultural biases facing those with mental illnesses, community size is another factor that reinforces stigma. In smaller communities, individuals with mental health needs are more likely to be assigned pejorative labels such as "crazy," primarily due to the fact that they are more "visible" than those in larger urban areas. This stigma may prevent those who need services from seeking them, due to fears that their confidentiality will be violated and the community will label them as "different." Social isolation is also a potential problem facing rural populations in need of mental health services, and an additional consequence of stigma.

Additional information is needed to understand the extent to which rural and urban mental health consumers differ in their utilization of mental health services. There is much discussion in the literature about what constitutes "urban" and "rural" relative to population density, proximity to metropolitan areas, and various psychological components of urban and rural life. While operational definitions vary along these dimensions (Nebraska Center for Rural Health Research, 1998), the University of Missouri's Office of Social and Economic Data Analysis (OSEDA) classifies counties throughout the State based upon the U.S. Census Bureau's definitions (U.S. Census Bureau, 2002). We used those areas classified as "metropolitan" by OSEDA to define "urban" in this study, and those listed as "non-metropolitan" to define "rural" (OSEDA, 2001). We felt these definitions of urban and rural best fit the need to identify counties based not solely on population, but also on proximity to urban areas, geographic isolation, and rural cultural character.

RESEARCH QUESTIONS

We examined rural/urban differences in mental health service utilization by answering three key questions. First, what is the accessibility of services to consumers in rural and (versus?) urban areas, as measured by the report of barriers such as housing, transportation, finances, and dual diagnoses? Second, what is their perception of the level of usefulness of services? Last, within the context that greater utilization and higher satisfaction with services indicate service acceptability, what is the level of service use and satisfaction?

To answer these questions, we examine rural/urban differences in accessibility, usefulness of services, and acceptability of services. While there are limitations to using consumer satisfaction scales as a measure of acceptability (Stallard, 1996; Campbell, 1999; Richard, 2000), they provide insights into consumers' perceptions of the differences in rural and urban mental health service utilization. Those insights also, in turn, have implications for the direction of rural mental health policy and for further research in this area. Moreover, our findings have special utility for advocates concerned about having an impact on state and local policy that ensures high quality services for individuals with severe mental illness in rural areas.

METHODOLOGY

Sample and Data Collection

The target population included all individuals who receive community-based services in the State of Missouri. From this population, a criterion sample of 311 individuals was identified for participation in the study. Rural and urban sample members were identified in mental health centers, self-help groups, social events for mental health consumers, and community meetings during a four-month period of 2002. This criterion sampling method delimited the study to a sample that could provide rich information regarding the extent to which residence in rural or urban counties mediates access to professional mental health services (Isaac & Michael, 1995, p. 224). Further, this sampling strategy was used to compensate for the lack of a sampling frame from which to randomly select mental health consumers in the State of Missouri.

A paper-and-pencil survey was administered to all respondents in the study. The researchers trained data collectors to administer the questionnaire to individuals or small groups of participants, depending on the information processing capacity of each participant. Data collectors, including both mental health consumers and professionals, were directed to self-help group meetings, community meetings, mental health centers, and recreational activities for mental health consumers in all regions of the state where such groups/meetings were held. Each participant had the ability to understand and answer the questions. At the beginning of each survey, the data collectors explained the purpose and format of the survey, emphasizing the confidentiality of all information collected. All participants signed a detailed informed consent form, and all responses were completely voluntary and anonymous.

Measures

The survey questionnaire used to collect data in this study was developed using a panel of experts. The members of the panel included a representative from each of the following communities/agencies/institutions: mental health consumers: Missouri Protection and Advocacy Services; the National Alliance for the Mentally Ill in Missouri; the Missouri Institute of Mental Health; and the University of Missouri's School of Social Work. All of these representatives assessed the face validity of the instrument and found it to be strong. Six measures were used to assess mental health services with respect to (1) accessibility relative to barriers, (2) availability, (3) affordability, (4) acceptability, (5) usefulness, and (6) satisfaction. In order to measure usefulness of services, a 5-point response format was used, which ranged from 1(least useful) to 5 (most useful). A dichotomous response format (yes/no) was used to measure accessibility, availability and acceptability of services.

To measure level of satisfaction with services, the Client Satisfaction Questionaire-8 (CSQ-8) was selected for use in the study primarily because it is simply worded, easily understood, brief, and applicable to a variety of settings (Attkisson, 1987). It was also chosen for its technical qualities (Campbell, 1999); it is normed with similar populations and has good construct validity, as well as excellent internal consistency (alphas = .86 − .94). Cronbach's alpha was .93 in this sample. The CSQ-8 consists of 8 individual items rated on a 5-point Likert-response format. Items and their response format included the following. *Quality of services*, measuring the degree of quality of services respondents received, ranged from 1(low quality) to 5 (high quality). *Degree of receiving wanted services* ranged from 1 (not at all pleased) to 5 (very pleased). *Degree of meeting my needs* ranged from 1 (do not meet my needs) to 5 (meet my needs very much). *Degree of recommending the services* ranged from 1 (do not recommend) to 5 (highly recommend). *Degree of satisfaction with the amount of help* ranged from 1 (not at all satisfied) to 5 (very satisfied). *Usefulness of services to deal with problems* ranged from 1 (not help at all) to 5 (helped a great deal). *Degree of seeking the same services* ranged from 1 (will not seek the same services) to 5 (will very much seek the same services). *Overall satisfaction with the services* ranged from 1 (not at all satisfied) to 5 (very satisfied).

Data Analyses

Chi-square and t-tests were used to explore group differences in the areas of demographic information, accessibility relative to barriers, availability, affordability, acceptability, usefulness, and satisfaction with services, with a specific focus on comparing those residing in rural and urban communities. All statistical tests are bivariate.

RESULTS

Demographic Differences Between Urban/Rural Groups

The results in Table 1 show that the sample approximates the racial diversity of the state and has good geographic and demographic representation of the state. The sample tends to be somewhat undereducated, not married, quite impoverished, and is more urban than rural. Overall, females and males comprised approximately 51 percent and 49 percent of participants, respectively. The majority of the sample (78%) reported they had at least high school diploma. Annual income categories included two hundred twenty-four individuals reporting under $8,001 (73.4%), sixty-eight reporting between $8,001-$20,000 (22.3%), and thirteen individuals reporting over $20,000 (4.3%), indicating that about the majority of the participants are financially poor.

There were statistically significant differences between two groups in age and ethnicity. In terms of age, sixty-one percent of rural respondents were older than 36-years-old, whereas about seventy-six percent of respondents were older than 36-years-old, showing that urban respondents were older than rural respondents. Compared with respondents in rural areas, the majority of urban respondents (93.6%) were Caucasians. Demographic characteristics are shown in Table 1 for respondents in both urban and rural areas.

Accessibility Relative to Barriers

Dual diagnosis, housing, transportation, and funding/financial resources were the barriers used in this study to reflect accessibility to services. More urban consumers perceived that housing was a barrier than

TABLE 1. Comparison of Demographic Characteristics by Residence

Variable	Urban (n = 216)	Rural (n = 95)	Total (n = 311)	Missouri State	Test Statistics χ^2
Age (%)					11.20*
18-21 years	1.8	6.3	3.2	5.9	
22-35 years	21.8	32.7	25.1	17.0	
36-50 years	51.4	34.7	46.3	22.9	
More than 50 years	25.0	26.3	25.4	28.9	
Gender (%)					1.79
Female	48.6	56.8	51.0	51.4	
Male	51.4	43.2	49.0	48.6	
Ethnicity (%)					13.34*
Caucasian	79.6	93.6	83.9	84.4	
African American	12.0	1.1	8.7	11.2	
Native American	3.7	4.3	3.9	0.4	
Hispanic/Latino	2.3	1.0	1.9	2.1	
Asian American	0.5	0.0	0.3	1.1	
Other	1.9	0.0	1.3	0.8	
Marital Status (%)					2.69
Single	55.8	50.0	54.0	24.8	
Married	9.8	9.6	9.7	55.5	
Separated	6.0	6.4	6.1	1.8	
Divorced	21.9	29.7	24.4	10.8	
Widowed	6.5	4.3	5.8	7.1	
Education (%)					1.86
Some high school	21.4	22.6	21.8	18.6	
High school diploma	41.2	47.3	43.0	32.7	
Some college	23.1	19.4	22.0	21.9	
College graduate	7.4	6.5	7.1	14.0	
Above college graduate	6.9	4.2	6.1	21.6	
Annual income (%)					2.69
Under $8,001	71.6	77.7	73.4	10.1	
$8,001 to $20,000	23.2	20.2	22.3	21.6	
$20,001 to $30,000	3.8	1.1	3.0	14.4	
Over $30,000	1.4	1.0	1.3	53.9	

*$p < .05$.

did rural consumers ($\chi^2 = 5.22$, $p < .05$). There were no significant differences in the perceptions of rural and urban consumers regarding dual diagnosis, housing, and transportation.

Availability of Services

As can be seen in Table 2, the results of Chi-square analysis on availability of services have been summarized. On a scale measuring overall availability of 12 services, urban consumers perceived greater availabil-

TABLE 2. Comparison for Perceived Availability of Services by Residence

Services	Urban		Rural		Test Statistics
	N	%	N	%	χ^2
Crisis services	174	92.1	84	94.4	0.49
Outreach–homeless	100	55.6	27	38.6	5.82*
Psychotherapy	180	89.6	72	82.8	2.56
Vocational services	159	81.5	73	85.9	0.79
Clubhouses	194	93.7	50	56.2	60.57***
Dual diagnosis group	153	81.0	41	50.6	25.80***
Maintenance level	179	89.9	60	73.2	12.86***
Group homes	141	72.7	60	71.4	0.05
Education	138	72.3	66	78.6	1.52
Mental health education	172	87.3	67	79.8	2.64
Transportation	181	88.3	66	79.5	3.73
Housing	189	93.6	80	94.1	0.03

*p < .05; ***p < .001.

ity of services (M = 9.2., SD = 2.65) than did rural consumers (M = 8.0, SD = 2.96) (t = −3.49, p < .001). Urban residents were significantly more aware of clubhouses (p < .001), dual diagnosis groups (p < .001), maintenance supports (p < .001), and outreach for the homeless (p < .05) in their communities than were rural consumers.

Affordability of Services

No difference was found between urban and rural residents on a bivariate measure of yearly income (Low = $8,000 or less per year; High = $8,001 or more per year). Further, no differences were found in those who pay for their services with Medicaid/Medicare/or a combination of both compared to those who pay with private insurance, self-pay, or use other means to pay between urban and rural residents.

Acceptability in Terms of Use of Services

In terms of overall use of twelve services, urban consumers used greater numbers of services (M = 5.9, SD = 2.4) than did rural consumers (M = 4.4, SD = 3.1; t = −4.73, p < .001). Chi square analysis showed that urban consumers utilized clubhouses, dual diagnosis groups, education about mental health, maintenance supports, and transportation more frequently than did rural consumers.

Usefulness of Services

Table 3 summarizes the results of t-tests on usefulness of services. Urban residents expressed significantly higher levels of usefulness of services, such as clubhouses (p < .01), maintenance supports (p < .01), and education (p < .01) than rural consumers.

Satisfaction with Services

As can be seen in Table 4, results of t-tests showed that urban consumers were significantly more satisfied with services than were their rural counterparts. There were significant group differences in all areas except in consumers' perceptions that the services they received helped them deal with their problems. Thus, urban consumers were more likely to have higher levels of satisfaction with services than were rural consumers.

In summary, the results of the study answer questions regarding the differences between rural and urban mental health service utilization. The findings support the study's expectations that rural consumers have less accessibility and availability to services, are less able to afford services, and are less accepted in their communities than are urban consumers.

TABLE 3. Comparison for Usefulness of Services by Residence

Services	Urban			Rural			Test Statistics
	N	M	SD	N	M	SD	t
Crisis services	77	3.78	1.43	37	3.35	1.42	−1.50
Outreach–homeless	22	3.82	1.33	6	3.17	1.72	−1.00
Psychotherapy	122	4.25	1.09	46	3.87	1.53	−1.78
Vocational services	88	3.86	1.27	40	3.63	1.41	−0.95
Clubhouses	179	4.48	0.95	29	3.83	1.47	−3.15**
Dual diagnosis group	62	3.71	1.51	9	3.78	1.48	−0.13
Maintenance level	154	4.41	0.97	34	3.88	1.41	−2.62**
Group homes	63	3.63	1.53	23	2.91	1.59	−1.92
Education	52	4.27	1.01	17	3.06	1.71	−3.56**
Mental health education	126	4.40	0.89	42	4.24	1.23	−0.91
Transportation	137	4.52	1.00	40	4.20	1.36	−1.62
Housing	114	4.47	1.03	51	4.33	1.19	−0.77

**p < .01.

TABLE 4. Comparison for Level of Service Satisfaction by Residence

Variable	Urban (n = 216)		Rural (n = 95)		Total (n = 311)		t test
	M	SD	M	SD	M	SD	
Quality of services you received	4.34	0.96	4.03	1.13	4.24	1.02	−2.40*
Received the services you wanted	4.28	1.04	3.83	1.22	4.14	1.11	−3.19**
Services received meet your needs	4.26	0.98	3.91	1.08	4.16	1.02	−2.74**
Recommend the services you received to a friend	4.50	0.89	4.11	1.23	4.38	1.02	−2.99**
Satisfied with amount of help received	4.32	1.03	3.83	1.23	4.17	1.12	−3.53***
Services received have helped deal with problems	4.20	1.05	3.97	1.13	4.13	1.08	−1.70
What extent will you seek same services if necessary	4.36	1.00	4.05	1.21	4.26	1.08	−2.93**
Overall satisfaction with services received	4.34	0.96	3.97	1.11	4.23	1.02	−2.27*

*p < .05; **p < .01; ***p < .001.

DISCUSSION AND CONCLUSIONS

Findings in most service utilization research show differences in rural and urban mental health service utilization related to service accessibility, availability, affordability, and acceptability. This study only marginally supports the study expectation that there are rural and urban differences in accessibility. Specifically, urban consumers were more likely than rural consumers to identify housing as a barrier to services, which is likely tied to the greater prevalence of homelessness among urban consumers.

The most important findings in this study were that rural consumers perceived that fewer services were available to them, used fewer services, and were less satisfied with services. The findings in this study failed to support prior evidence that there are rural and urban consumer differences in income and rates of public health care benefits. These findings were not surprising in light of the large pockets of poverty found in Kansas City and St. Louis, Missouri's two largest urban areas. Taken together, these findings support the idea that rurality is negatively associated with both service availability and acceptability.

Some limitations to the study should be noted. They include those related to accessibility issues, mental health diagnosis and sampling. The following illustrate some of these limitations. Accessibility issues, such as distance from home to mental health services and geographic isolation are particularly important given the emphasis of the Americans With Disabilities Act on access to care (Rinere & Morris, 1997). Future studies should examine these as possible barriers in addition to those studied here.

The mental health diagnoses of participating consumers were not obtainable in the current study. It is difficult to know how important this variable might be. Findings in previous research show that the prevalence rate of many disorders is similar in rural and urban regions (see NIMH, 2000). With these findings in mind, it is likely that a diagnostic variable in this study would have had relatively little impact on the relationship between rurality and mental health service utilization.

Finally, it should be noted that this study did not employ random sampling. Missouri, however, is often referred to as the "political weathervane, and almost exactly mirrors the nation" (Public Broadcasting System, 2000). This is primarily due to its balance of rural and urban dwellers, as well as its racial mix–84% white, 14% black, and 2% other. Our sample closely approximates the demographics of the state, allowing us some confidence in the applicability of our findings.

IMPLICATIONS FOR POLICY, PRACTICE, AND RESEARCH

Mental health policy advocates should focus on the key issues for rural mental health consumers, especially lack of available services and cultural characteristics of communities that prevent those who need services from seeking them. There is evidence that mental health programs with a rural focus can succeed in training more workers for these shortage areas (Mohatt & Kirwan, 1995). Yet, too many mental health programs are neglecting a "generalist mental health practitioner" model that allows the flexibility of skills necessary for the multiple roles required in rural settings. More federal stipends are needed to initiate rural mental health training programs, with a requirement that newly educated professionals begin practice in a federally designated rural shortage area.

In light of the fact that general medical practitioners see the majority of individuals with mental health problems in rural areas, physicians in rural areas need to be better educated about mental health screening, diagnosis, treatment, and continuing care (MRHRC, 1997). Unfortunately, there are few opportunities for physicians in rural areas to consult with trained mental health personnel. Continuing education and consultation opportunities in mental health care for primary care physicians could include:

in-service trainings, assigning mental health professionals to travel between rural areas to consult with general practitioners, and distance-education via the Internet.

Telemedicine is the state-of-the-art technique to address availability/accessibility problems in rural mental health (NIMH, 2000). The focus of many of these programs, however, is to ensure access to psychiatrists for purposes of medication prescription and monitoring. As a result, programs fail to address the needs of those who are typically responsible for the day-to-day care of persons with mental illness, especially social workers, psychologists, and psychiatric nurses. By neglecting the consultative and educational needs of those mental health professionals who supply day-to-day care, ADA prescriptions for access to services for those with mental disabilities and those in need of psychiatric rehabilitation (Granger & Gill, 2000) are affected. The rural consumer who can access the psychiatrist by phone for prescription medication, but who has no access to a supportive social worker or case manager will likely not remain adequately housed and/or stabilized in the community. Given the results of this study–that rural mental health consumers perceive less available, less frequently used and less satisfactory services than those in urban areas–it appears that continuing support for mental health professionals is important to building an effective rural mental health workforce. While a regression analysis in a previous study using this same data showed that participation in self-help services predicted the greatest amount of variance in consumer scores on ratings of satisfaction, the interaction between urban/rural residence and participation in self-help services was not explored (Hodges, Markward, Keele, & Evans, 2003). Future research should explore how these two constructs co-vary, and to what extent participation in self-help services is affected by urban vs. rural residence.

Last, further research seems warranted to identify the link between perceived service availability and service satisfaction, especially if perceptions of rural consumers in some way mediate service satisfaction/use. Although perceived availability of services and urban residence predicted service satisfaction in this study, the two variables co-varied, indicating the need to explore the link between rurality and awareness of mental health services. Within the context that *actual* service availability in rural areas is lacking, further research also is needed to determine how traditional rural values of self-reliance, service awareness, and service use are linked, if at all. Even if an adequate supply of mental health services and professionals existed in rural areas, these cultural characteristics might prevent their utilization.

REFERENCES

Attkisson, C. C. (1987). Client satisfaction questionnaire (CSQ-8). In K. Corcoran, & J. Fischer (Eds.), *Measures for clinical practice: A sourcebook* (pp. 120-122). New York: The Free Press.

Bushy, A. (1997). *Mental health and substance abuse: Challenges in providing services to rural clients.* School of Nursing, University of Central Florida. Report available online at the Missouri Institute of Mental Health's Policy Information Exchange: *http://www.mimh.edu/mimhweb/pie/database/GetArticle.asp?value=596*

Campbell, J. (1999). *Exemplary practices for measuring consumer satisfaction: A review of the literature, Part One, Two, & Three.* Missouri Institute of Mental Health, Policy Information Exchange (PIE). Accessible at: *http://www.mimh.edu/mimhweb/pie/database/GetArticle.asp?value=1602*

Granger, B., & Gill, P. (2000). Strategies for assisting people with psychiatric disabilities to assert their ADA rights and arrange job accommodations. *Psychiatric Rehabilitation Skills, 4*(1), 120-135.

Hartley, D., Bird, D., & Dempsey, P. (1999). Mental health and substance abuse. In *Rural Health in the United States.* New York: Oxford University Press.

Hodges, J.Q., Markward, M., Keele, C., & Evans, C. (2003). Use of self-help services and consumer satisfaction with professional mental health services. *Psychiatric Services, 54*(8), 1161-1163.

Hoyt, D.R., Conger, R.D., Valde, J.G., & Weihs, K. (1997). Psychological distress and help seeking in rural America. *American Journal of Community Psychology, 25*(4), 449-470.

Isaac, S., & Michael, W.B. (1995). *Handbook in Research and Evaluation.* Educational and Industrial Testing Services: San Diego, CA.

Maine Rural Health Research Center (MRHRC) (1997). *Research & Policy Brief: Why do rural Medicaid beneficiaries with depression use fewer mental health services: Is supply the issue?* March, 1997. Available online at the Missouri Institute of Mental Health's Policy Information Exchange at: *http://www.mimh.edu/mimhweb/pie/database/GetArticle.asp?value=2939*

Maine Rural Health Research Center (MRHRC) (1999a). *Best practices in rural Medicaid managed behavioral health: 1, Measuring & Monitoring Access.* Hartley, D. (Ed.), Edmund S. Muskie School of Public Service. Available online at the Missouri Institute of Mental Health Policy Information Exchange: *http://www.mimh.edu/mimhweb/pie/database/GetArticle.asp?value=2882*

Maine Rural Health Research Center (MRHRC) (1999b). *Best practices in rural Medicaid managed behavioral health: 4, Consumer issues.* Hartley, D. (Ed.), Edmund S. Muskie School of Public Service. Available online at the Missouri Institute of Mental Health Policy Information Exchange: *http://www.mimh.edu/*

Mohatt, D.F. (1997). *Access to mental health services in frontier America: Letter to the field No. 4.* Nebraska Department of Health and Human Services.

Mohatt, D.F., & Kirwan, D.M. (Eds.) (1995). *Meeting the challenge: Model programs in rural mental health.* Office of Rural Health Policy. Wood River, IL: National Association for Rural Mental Health. Available online at the Missouri

Institute of Mental Health's Policy Information Exchange: *http://www.mimh.edu/ mimhweb/pie/database/GetArticle.asp?value=131*

National Institute of Mental Health (NIMH) (2000). *Rural mental health research at the National Institute of Mental Health*. Fact sheet, Office of Communications and Public Liaison, September 2000.

National Rural Health Association (NRHA) (1999). *Mental health in rural America: An issue paper presented by the National Rural Health Association–May 1999*. Available online at: *http://www.nrharural.org/dc/issuepapers/ipaper14. html*

Nebraska Center for Rural Health Research (NCRHR) (1998). *Rural/urban definitions: Alternatives and numbers by state*. Project Report 98-1, The National Rural Health Association, Rural Health Policy Board. Available online at the Missouri Institute of Mental Health's Policy Information Exchange at: *http://www.mimh. edu/mimhweb/pie/database/GetArticle.asp?value=2131*

Office of Social and Economic Data Analysis (OSEDA) (2001). *Trendletter, April 2001: Missouri's 2000 Population*. University of Missouri, Columbia. Available at: *http://www.oseda.missouri.edu/trendltr/yr2001/census2000.html*

Public Broadcasting System (PBS) (2000). Website: "The choice 2000: Why Missouri?" Available at: *http://www.pbs.org/wgbh/pages/frontline/shows/choice 2000/ undecided/missouri.html*

Richard, M.A. (2000). A discrepancy model for measuring consumer satisfaction with rehabilitation services. *The Journal of Rehabilitation, 66*(14), 37-49.

Rinere, V., & Morris, J. (1997). A model for stage agency compliance with the ADA: Ensuring access for people with mental illnesses. *Psychiatric Rehabilitation Journal, 21*(2), 177-180.

Schurman, R.A., Kramer, R.D., & Mitchell, J.B. (1985). The hidden mental health network. *Archives of General Psychiatry, 42*, 89-94.

Stallard, P. (1996). The role and use of consumer satisfaction surveys in mental health services. *Journal of Mental Health, 5*(4), 333-348.

Stefl, M.E., & Prosperi, D.C. (1985). Barriers to mental health service utilization. *Community Mental Health Journal, 21*(3), 167-178.

U.S. Census Bureau (2002). *Census 2000 Geographic Terms and Concepts*. Available on-line at: *http://www.census.gov/geo/www/tiger/glossry2.pdf*

Wagenfeld, M.O., Goldsmith, H.F., Stiles, D., & Manderscheid, R.W. (1988). Inpatient mental health services in metropolitan and non-metropolitan counties. *Journal of Rural Community Psychology, 9*(2), 13-28.

Wagenfeld, M.O., Murray, J.D., Mohatt, D.F. & DeBruyn, J. (Eds.). (1994). *Mental health and rural America: An overview and annotated bibliography 1978-1993*. Washington, DC: U.S. Government Printing Office.

An Analysis
of the Americans
With Disabilities Act (ADA)
in the Twenty-First Century

John T. Pardeck

SUMMARY. In this paper, the author overviews the key components of the ADA. A discussion is offered on why and how persons with disabilities are discriminated against. The standard stereotypes often heard about persons with disabilities are offered. Critical United States Supreme Court decisions are presented; these decisions have greatly limited the power of the ADA in protecting the rights of persons with disabilities. Even though the United States Supreme Court has narrowed the impact of the ADA in American life, a number of Equal Employment Opportunity Commission (EEOC) cases are presented, suggesting this federal agency is attempting to protect persons with disabilities against discrimination. The final part of the

John T. Pardeck, PhD, LCSW, was formerly Professor of Social Work, School of Social Work, Southwest Missouri State University, Springfield, MO 65804. He is now deceased.

[Haworth co-indexing entry note]: "An Analysis of the Americans With Disabilities Act (ADA) in the Twenty-First Century." Pardeck, John T. Co-published simultaneously in *Journal of Social Work in Disability & Rehabilitation* (The Haworth Social Work Practice Press, an imprint of The Haworth Press, Inc.) Vol. 4, No. 1/2, 2005, pp. 121-151; and: *Disability Issues for Social Workers and Human Services Professionals in the Twenty-First Century* (ed: John W. Murphy, and John T. Pardeck) The Haworth Social Work Practice Press, an imprint of The Haworth Press, Inc., 2005, pp. 121-151. Single or multiple copies of this article are available for a fee from The Haworth Document Delivery Service [1-800-HAWORTH, 9:00 a.m. - 5:00 p.m. (EST). E-mail address: docdelivery@haworthpress.com].

paper deals with the topic of advocacy; advocacy may well be one of the most effective tools to help insure that the rights of people with disabilities are protected in the 21st century. *[Article copies available for a fee from The Haworth Document Delivery Service: 1-800-HAWORTH. E-mail address: <docdelivery@haworthpress.com> Website: <http://www.HaworthPress.com>* © *2005 by The Haworth Press, Inc. All rights reserved.]*

KEYWORDS. ADA, persons with disabilities, disability discrimination, disability stereotypes, advocacy, court rulings

On July 26, 1990, President Bush senior signed the Americans With Disabilities Act (ADA) into law. This legislation is referred to as the "emancipation proclamation for the disabled" because of its great importance to members of American society with disabilities. It covers 43 million Americans with disabling conditions. These disabilities stretch across a broad spectrum of types and severity. The ADA has significant implications for all citizens, not only those with disabilities. The ADA also has significance for how social work agencies and other systems operate. For example, for local governments, changes have been required in countless ordinances, building codes and policies. Public social work agencies must also make these changes. For private industry, including the for profit social work agencies, many changes have been required for compliance with the ADA. These include hiring procedures, job restructuring, work schedules, training materials and equipment used, and other factors affecting persons with disabilities working in or coming in contact with the private sector. In essence, the ADA has profound implications for all aspects of American life including the profession of social work (Pardeck, 1998).

THE AMERICANS WITH DISABILITIES ACT

The ADA is grounded in a philosophy that views unequal treatment of persons with disabilities as a violation of their human rights. The ADA is based on the position that persons with disabilities have not received the same treatment as others, and that it is the responsibility of the state to affirm or re-affirm those rights through judicial and legislative actions. The ADA views people with disabilities as having intrinsic worth and dignity. However, there is also a utilitarian theme that guides the ADA; for example, employers must make reasonable accommodations to assist the person with a disability in the work place. In other words the cost for accommodating the person with a disability cannot necessarily outweigh the benefits. This utilitarian view always stresses the practicality and cost effectiveness of programs (Pardeck, 1998).

Findings Supporting Need for the ADA

The ADA (P.L. Law 101-336, 1990) was signed into law based on the following findings:

1. There are 43 million Americans who have one or more physical or mental disabilities.
2. Historically society has tended to isolate and segregate the disabled.
3. Discrimination in the areas of employment, housing, public accommodations, transportation, and education has been an incredible deterrent in the implementation of the rights of the disabled.
4. Discrimination on the basis of disability frequently had no legal recourse.
5. Individuals with disabilities are intentionally excluded by architectural, transportation or communication barriers, and practices that result in lesser opportunities.
6. People with disabilities as a group occupy inferior status and are disadvantaged socially, vocationally, economically, and educationally.
7. Individuals with disabilities are a distinct and insular minority who have been faced with restrictions and limitations and subjected to unequal treatment.
8. The nation's proper goals should be to assure equality of opportunity, full participation, independent living, and economic self-sufficiency.
9. The continued existence of unfair and unnecessary discrimination against the disabled denies opportunity to compete, and costs the United States billions of dollars in unnecessary expenses resulting from dependency and nonproductively.

Purposes of the ADA

There are four purposes of the ADA based upon the nine findings:

1. To provide a national mandate to eliminate discrimination against individuals with disabilities.

2. To provide an enforceable standard addressing discrimination.
3. To ensure that the federal government will play a central role in enforcing these standards.
4. To involve congressional authority in order to address the major areas of discrimination faced by people with disabilities.

There are five major Titles under the ADA. The definition of "disability" established in the Rehabilitation Act of 1973 is adopted in the ADA. This definition is as follows: Disability means a physical or mental impairment that substantially limits one or more of the major life activities of an individual, a record of such impairment, or being regarded as having such impairment.

Under this definition, disabilities include the following kinds of problems–mobility impairments, sensory impairments, mental retardation, and other physical and mental impairments including hidden disabilities such as cancer, diabetes, epilepsy, heart disease, and mental illness. Individuals who have a history of these disabilities but are no longer disabled, or who have been incorrectly classified as having a disability, or who do not have a disability but who are treated or perceived by others as having a disability, are protected by the ADA (Pardeck, 1998).

Major Titles of the ADA

Title I. Discrimination Regarding Employment. This Title defines and describes how employers are prohibited from discriminating against a qualified individual with a disability in all terms and conditions of employment. This Title has the greatest importance for employee selection.

Title II. Public Services. This Title prohibits discrimination and increases the accessibility of persons with disabilities to programs run by state and local governments. For the field of social work this includes public social work agencies, colleges and universities. This title also requires that public transportation become accessible to people with disabilities.

Title III. Private Accommodations and Services. This Title requires that private businesses serving the public make their goods and services available to people with disabilities.

Title IV. The Telecommunications Title. This Title requires that telephone services be accessible to people with hearing and speech impairments by providing them with relay services. The relay service uses an operator as an intermediary communicator between the hearing person and the individual needing assistance.

Title V. Miscellaneous. This Title prohibits retaliation against an individual because of actions related to the Act, and provides information on the implementation of the ADA, the Rehabilitation Act of 1973, and state laws.

Title I (Employment)

The Rehabilitation Act of 1973 was the first significant national legislation to protect people with disabilities. The Rehabilitation Act, however, only covers those entities that receive federal contracts or subcontracts exceeding a certain dollar amount. The Rehabilitation Act has served as the model for the Americans With Disabilities Act including Title I of the ADA. In fact, the definition for a disability under the ADA was borrowed from the Rehabilitation Act (Pardeck, 1998).

Title I of the ADA covers all employers, both public and private, who employ 15 or more workers. Since employment discrimination has long been a problem for people with disabilities, the goal of Title I is to prevent this kind of discrimination (Pardeck, 1998).

Discrimination against people with disabilities occurs in many different forms in the workplace. Some of the discrimination is intentional; some is unintentional. Much of the discrimination against people with disabilities is a result of able people seeing the disabled as different from others. The media has portrayed people with disabilities as different and often this portrayal is in extremes. For example, some people with disabilities are viewed as extremely dependent; others are presented as super heroes such as Ironside from the famous television series about the lawyer who used a wheelchair. These extremes are often unrealistic and do not help the able better understand people with disabilities. As children, most people often experienced educational systems that segregated people with disabilities from others. This kind of segregation also extended into the workplace, for example, the placement of persons with disabilities in Sheltered Workshops. This kind of separation has increased our lack of awareness of the person with disabilities and their special needs. Segregation of people with disabilities from the able emphasizes the differences of people in the two groups and not their similarities. Segregation of people with disabilities in schools and the workplace has increased able persons' fears and discomfort with people who have disabilities (Pardeck, 1998).

Title I of the ADA is aimed at changing the historical patterns of excluding people with disabilities from the workplace. The objective of Title I is to place people with disabilities into meaningful employment and to offer them job opportunities that nondisabled people take for granted. Once people with disabilities have achieved greater integration into the workplace, many of the misconceptions about people with disabilities will be eliminated (Pardeck, 1998).

To comply with Title I, employers must make sure that the employee selection process is clearly understood by all employees. The requirements of the ADA in the area of employment must be provided to all employees. Employers must understand that the employment provisions of the ADA cover hiring, promotions, pay, firing, job training, benefits, and virtually all aspects of the workplace. National legislators recognized that they could not predict every possible form of employment discrimination, so they created a law that is broad and open to interpretation. An important component of Title I is defining who is protected and outlining the basic responsibilities of employers (Pardeck, 1998).

Employers must understand that Title I includes a definition for not only a disability under the law but also for what is meant by a qualified individual with a disability. A qualified individual with a disability under the employment provisions of the ADA is as follows (Equal Employment Opportunity Commission & U. S. Department of Justice, 1992):

> A qualified individual with a disability is a person who meets legitimate skill, experience, education, or other requirements of an employment position that s/he holds or seeks, and who can perform the "essential" functions of the position with or without reasonable accommodation. Requiring the ability to perform "essential" functions assures that an individual with a disability will not be considered unqualified simply because of inability to perform marginal or incidental job functions. (p. 2)

An employer must realize that if an individual is qualified to perform essential job functions except for limitations caused by a disability, the employer must consider whether the individual could perform these functions with a reasonable accommodation. If a written job description has been prepared in advance of advertising or interviewing applicants for a job, this will be considered as evidence, although not conclusive evidence, of the essential functions of the job (Pardeck, 1998).

Essential functions of a job include the fundamental duties required of a position. These qualifications include educational requirements, work experience, training levels, job skills, licensing and certification requirements, and other job related requirements determined by the employer (Pardeck, 1998).

Even though the ADA does not mandate it, employers should have a complete job description for all positions in an organization including those that the employer wishes to fill. The essential function of a job is the primary responsibilities of the position. Employers should list in writing any key duties for a position; these should become a part of the job description. Title I does not require employers to eliminate or make changes to core job duties or essential functions of the job for the person with a disability. However, every position typically has several tasks that are not vital to the position; these kinds of tasks are viewed as non-essential functions. Under the ADA, an employer cannot refuse to hire a person with a disability because of their inability to do a nonessential task (Pardeck, 1998).

Title I emphasizes that an organization has every right to hire the most qualified individual. Obviously, the most qualified individual is the one who can best perform the essential functions of the job, with or without accommodations. It is the employer's responsibility to determine these essential functions. Employers should be prepared, however, to provide reasonable accommodations to help the person with a disability perform a job (Pardeck, 1998).

Essential functions of a job are related to the definition of a qualified individual with a disability. A qualified person with a disability is one who meets all of the qualifications of a job including but not limited to educational requirements, work experience, training skills, and licensing and certification requirements. If a person with a disability applies for a position, an employer must determine if these essential functions can be performed with or without reasonable accommodations. When considering individuals for a position, it is critical for the employer to apply hiring criteria consistently to all applicants including the able and persons with disabilities. If a person with a disability is the most qualified person for a position, that person should be offered the position. This is equally true for the able person (Pardeck, 1998).

A reasonable accommodation is also an important aspect of Title I as well as other Titles under the ADA. A reasonable accommodation is a modification or adjustment for a position, which helps a qualified individual with a disability perform the tasks of a job. The employer can accommodate both the essential functions and the nonessential functions of a position (Pardeck, 1998).

Title II (Public Services)

This Title of the ADA prohibits discrimination against persons with disabilities in all services, programs, and activities provided or made available by state or local government. Many state and local governments were prohibited from discriminating against persons with disabilities prior to the ADA under Section 504 of the Rehabilitation Act of 1973. Section 504 prohibits discrimination on the basis of disability in any programs and activities that receive a set amount of federal funds. Title II of the ADA extends the nondiscrimination requirements of Section 504 to the activities of all state and local governments, regardless of whether they receive any federal support. Title II has two subtitles, A and B. Subtitle A covers all activities of state and local governments other than public transit. Subtitle B deals with the provision of publicly funded transit (Pardeck, 1998).

Activities Covered Under Title II. Title II covers every type of state or local government activity or program. In employment, state and local governments cannot discriminate against job applicants and employees with disabilities regardless of the number of people they employ (Pardeck, 1998).

Title III (Public Accommodations and Services)

Title III of the ADA covers private accommodations and services. Title III requires that private businesses serving the public make their goods and services available to people with disabilities. Titles II and III are very similar in scope; however, Title II covers state and local governments, where Title III covers private entities.

Titles IV and V

Title IV of the ADA requires that telephone services be accessible to people with hearing and speech impairments by providing them with relay services.

Title V prohibits retaliation against an individual because of actions related to the Act, and provides information on the implementation of the ADA, the Rehabilitation Act of 1973, and state laws.

DISCRIMINATION ON THE BASIS OF DISABILITY

Harrison and Gilbert (1992) report findings from various testimonies made by individuals and representatives of various organizations concerning the need for the passage of the ADA. For example, Timothy Cook of the National Disability Action Center testified (Harrison and Gilbert, 1992):

> As Rosa Parks taught us, and as the Supreme Court ruled thirty-five years ago in Brown v. Board of Education, segregation "affects one's heart and mind in ways that may never be undone. Separate but equal is inherently unequal." (p. 10)

Others testified that discrimination also included exclusion, or denial of benefits, services, or other opportunities that are as effective and meaningful as those provided to others. Furthermore, discrimination results from actions or inactions that discriminate by effect as well as by intention. Under these circumstances, discrimination includes the lack of access to buildings, standards and criteria, and practices based on thoughtlessness or indifference, that discriminate against persons with disabilities (Harrison and Gilbert, 1992).

Testimony presented by Judith Heumann of the World Institute on Disability illustrated several forms of discrimination well known to people with disabilities. Heumann stated (Harrison and Gilbert, 1992):

> When I was 5 my mother proudly pushed my wheelchair to our local public school, where I was promptly refused admission because the principal ruled that I was a fire hazard. I was forced to go into home instruction, receiving one hour of education twice a week for 3 1/2 years. My entrance into mainstream society was blocked by discrimination and segregation. Segregation was not only on an institutional level but also acted as an obstruction to social integration. As a teenager, I could not travel with friends on the bus because it was not accessible. At my graduation from high school, the principal attempted to prevent me from accepting an award in a ceremony on stage simply because I was in a wheelchair. (p. 11)

Other testimony supporting Ms. Heumann's experiences reported that having a history of a disability and being regarded as having a disability or even associating with people with disabilities often resulted in discrimination. Discrimination also included the effects of a person's disability on others. For example, a child with Down's Syndrome was refused admittance to a zoo because the zoo keeper felt the child would upset the chimpanzees. In another case a cerebral palsied child was denied admission to school because the teacher claimed his physical appearance produced a nauseating effect on his classmates. During Senate testimony Senator Mondale described a case in which a woman crippled by arthritis was denied a job not because she could not do the work, but because college trustees felt normal students should not see her. Finally, a number of individuals testified that they were denied jobs because they had AIDS, were former cancer victims, had epilepsy, and other serious illnesses (Harrison and Gilbert, 1992).

Major public opinion polls such as the Harris poll found that by almost any definition, people with disabilities are uniquely underprivileged and disadvantaged. They are much poorer, much less educated and have less social life and lower levels of self-satisfaction than other Americans (Harrison and Gilbert, 1992).

All of the data and testimony gathered by the Congress that resulted in the passage of the ADA found that persons with disabilities experience discrimination in virtually every aspect of American life. Individuals with disabilities experience staggering levels of unemployment and poverty. Two-thirds of all people with disabilities between the ages of 16 and 64 are not working at all, yet a large majority of those not working want to work. Sixty-six percent of working-aged people with disabilities not working wanted a job. What emerged from the research conducted by the Congress was that persons with disabilities were one of the most oppressed minority groups in the United States (Harrison and Gilbert, 1992).

MODELS FOR DEFINING DISABILITY

The various models for understanding and defining disability are grounded in a number of cultural traditions. One tradition in the United States has been to view the concept of disability through a moral model. The moral model has also influenced the development of the medical model which emerged in the 1900s. The medical model has had a significant influence on how various helping professions assess and treat persons with disabilities (Pardeck, 2002).

The moral model views persons with disabilities as being at odds with the moral and spiritual order (Longmore, 1993). Longmore (1993) suggests that the moral model not only views persons with disabilities as being punished for wrong doing, but also implies that they are the cause of the disability. The ancient roots of the moral model can be found in the writings of the early Greeks (Pardeck, 2002); the Romans also endorsed this model (Pardeck, 2002). Both the Greeks and Romans at times abandoned their disabled or deformed children to die (Pardeck, 2002).

Judeo-Christianity has strong underpinnings of the moral model. Livenel (1982) reports that from the Middle Ages to the present, a tradition in Judeo-Christianity has been to view a disability as being a reflection of God's displeasure with a person. This tradition in Judeo-Christianity has linkages to ancient Greek and Roman cultures (Pardeck, 2002).

The medical model, a relatively new perspective, is grounded in the moral model. Both perspectives share one common belief, that persons with disabilities are flawed and must be changed or treated. The medical model obscures this view under the auspices of science, the moral model under the teachings of theology. The medical model defines persons with disabilities as having biological inadequacies; the moral model suggests that disabilities are caused by spiritual flaws. The goal of the medical model is to cure the person with a disability through various kinds of clinical interventions (Pardeck, 2002).

Jennic Marsh, a person with a disability who is an activist in the civil rights movement for people with disabilities succinctly describes the medical model's approach to disability as quoted in Mackelprang and Salsgiver (1999):

> I was barely human. One time, as a 14-year-old, I was paraded in front of a whole class of doctors so they could see my "abnormal gait." I was wearing only my panties. They would never have done that to a nondisabled girl but it was OK to parade me almost naked. And the crazy thing is, it wasn't until years later that I realized they had dehumanized me. (p. 39)

In contrast to the moral and medical models, the minority group model offers a dramatically different view of disability. The minority group model views a disability as a social construct that is no different from race or gender. Given this position, the limitations often associated with a disability are created by society not the person. An emerging philosophical and political view within the civil rights disability movement, the independent living movement, endorses this view. The independent living movement emerged from the turbulence of the 1960s. It challenges the traditional view of disability and argues that society creates and perpetuates how persons with disabilities are defined and treated. According to the independent living movement, society must change, not the person with a disability. The ADA is grounded in this notion. It will be argued in this chapter that the independent living movement employs some of the most effective strategies for promoting the minority group model of disability. The ADA provides the framework for helping to insure that these strategies are effective (Pardeck, 2002).

Stereotyping of Persons with Disabilities

The moral and medical models have greatly shaped society's perception of persons with disabilities; this perception is based on a number of stereotypes that are well established in American culture. The term ableism captures the essence of this phenomenon (Pardeck, 2002). Ableism is defined as the belief that people with disabilities are inferior to nondisabled people because they are different (Mackelprang and Salsgiver, 1999). Like racism, ableism is shaped by stereotypes that are often used to separate persons with disabilities from able persons. Stereotypes defining persons with disabilities include the following (Pardeck 2002):

1. Object of Pity–Viewing persons with disabilities as objects who merit the pity of the able world. This view endorses the notion that a disability may be worse than death.
2. Threat to Society–A belief that the person with a disability is a menace to society. Persons with developmental and emotional disabilities have a tendency to fall into the threat to society category. This stereotype reinforces the notion that persons with disabilities may hurt others if they are not controlled. This stereotype has lead to the institutionalization of persons with disabilities.
3. Perpetual Children–A belief that even though the person with a disability is an adult, he or she should be treated like a child. Unlike the nondisabled person, the person with a disability is not seen as going through the developmental life cycle. Given this belief, there are low expectations for persons with disabilities because they simply never grow up.

4. Curse From God–This view supports the notion that persons with disabilities are being punished by God because of their own sins or the sins of their parents. This stereotype produces guilt and shame for persons with disabilities and their families.
5. Freaks–A belief that dehumanizes persons with disabilities. An excellent example of this stereotype is developed in Victor Hugo's (1991) hunchback from Notre Dame, Quasimodo. Quasimodo's "ugliness" was equated with evil; he was made to feel evil and unimportant because of his appearance.

The above stereotypes have been used to segregate and discriminate against persons with disabilities. Prior to the passage of the ADA, many social institutions used the above stereotypes as justification for discrimination against a person because of his or her disability. For example, prior to the 1990s, an employer could simply fire an employee because the person was a cancer survivor. Such behavior is now a violation of the ADA. Cancer survivors, like many other persons with disabilities, are 5 times more likely to be fired or laid off than other employees (Arnold, 1999). Research also reports that up to 50 percent of cancer survivors feel they are discriminated against in the workplace because they had cancer (Arnold, 1999). Examples of why cancer survivors are confronted with job discrimination include the following beliefs and stereotypes (Pardeck, 1998):

1. Cancer survivors are viewed as having higher rates of absenteeism than other employees. This belief is not supported by fact.
2. Many employers have a traditional view of cancer; they simply think cancer means death. Often employers do not realize that many cancers can be cured or controlled.
3. Some employers discriminate against cancer survivors because they simply do not feel comfortable having them in the workplace. This is a common problem for people confronted with other kinds of disabilities.
4. Some employers feel that cancer survivors will drive their health care costs up. This belief is based on fiction, not fact.

The above beliefs about cancer survivors are very similar to the stereotypes often used to justify discrimination against other groups of persons with disabilities. The ADA is an important federal law that is helping to change these stereotypes (Pardeck, 2002).

RECENT SUPREME COURT RULINGS ON THE ADA

HIV Infection

Bragdon v. Abbott (524 U.S. 624, June 25, 1998) resulted in an important ruling by the United States Supreme Court concerning persons who have HIV infection. The Court ruled that a person with HIV infection even though it has not yet progressed to the so-called symptomatic phase is disabled under the ADA. The Court also affirmed that patients infected with HIV posed no direct threat to the health and safety of dentist. One could generalize this ruling to health care providers in general (Pardeck, 2001).

In the Bragdon v. Abbott case, Sidney Abbott, an HIV infected patient, seeking dental treatment from Dr. Randon Bragdon in 1994 disclosed her HIV infection on the patient registration form. Dr. Bragdon refused to treat her in his office. He did, however, offer to perform the dental treatment needed in a hospital facility. Ms. Abbott refused the treatment and filed a law suit against Dr. Bragdon alleging that Dr. Bragdon's refusal to treat her in his dental office was a violation of her civil rights under the ADA. A Federal court ruled that Ms. Abbott was discriminated against by Dr. Bragdon under the ADA. In 1998, the Supreme Court upheld the lower courts ruling (Pardeck, 2001).

Corrections

In the Pennsylvania Department of Corrections v. Yeskey (524 U.S. 206, June 15, 1998) the United States Supreme Court held that state prison systems must provide reasonable accommodations to prisoners under the ADA. Ronald R. Yeskey was an inmate sentence to serve 18 to 36 months in a Pennsylvania correctional facility. The sentencing court recommended that Mr. Yeskey be placed in Pennsylvania's Motivational Boot Camp for first-time offenders, completing the camp would have led to his release on parole in just six months. However, because of his medical history of hypertension, he was refused admission to the first-time offender's program. Mr. Yeskey alleged that exclusion from the Boot Camp because of his hypertension violated the ADA (Pardeck, 2001).

Mr. Yeskey filed suit in federal court against the Pennsylvania Correctional system. The Correctional system argued that prisoners are not protected under the ADA. The lower court ruled that Mr. Yeskey was discriminated under the ADA and that the Pennsylvania Correctional System violated Title II of the ADA which covers state run programs, services, and activities including prisons. The United States Supreme Court upheld the lower courts decision in 1998 (Pardeck, 2001).

Social Security Benefits (SSDI) and the ADA

In Cleveland v. Policy Management (526 U.S. 795, May 24, 1999) the United States Supreme Court reversed a lower federal court decision that held an applicant filing for or receiving SSDI does not automatically bar an individual from filing an ADA lawsuit. The plaintiff in this case, Carolyn Cleveland, was employed by Policy Management System Corporation in a position that required her to perform background checks on job applicants. She experienced a stroke in January 1994, the stroke impaired her concentration, language skills and memory. Several weeks after her stroke she filed an application for SSDI, in which she indicated that she was disabled and not able to work (Pardeck, 2001).

After filing for SSDI, her condition improved and she returned to work. Cleveland reported to the Social Security Administration that she had returned to work, her benefits application was then denied. Three months after returning to work, however, she was fired by her employer because she "could no longer do her job because of her condition." After termination, Cleveland asked the Social Security Administration to reconsider her SSDI application (Pardeck, 2001).

Cleveland was approved for SSDI benefits one year after her reapplication; she received benefits retroactive to the day of her stroke. A week before receiving her SSDI benefit award, however, she filed an ADA lawsuit contending that her employer terminated her without reasonably accommodating her disability by offering additional training and time to complete her work. A federal court ruled in favor of her employer. The lower court concluded that an application for or the receipt of SSDI benefits creates a rebuttable presumption that the claimant is not a qualified person with a disability under the ADA (Pardeck, 2001).

Cleveland's case was appealed to the United States Supreme Court. Addressing the similarities and differences between the Social Security Act and the ADA, the Supreme Court observed that both laws help individuals with disabilities in different ways. The Social Security Act provides monetary benefits to people who have a disability, while the ADA seeks to eliminate unwarranted discrimination against persons with disabilities. In other words, just because a person applies for or receives SSDI benefits does not automatically mean he or she loses ADA rights. Under the ADA, each case must be assessed on the case's own merits; this process was lost when the lower federal court ruled that Carolyn Cleveland could not file a law suit under the ADA because of her application for SSDI benefits (Pardeck, 2001).

Defining a Disability Under the ADA

During the summer of 1999 the United States Supreme Court attempted to help clarify the definition of a disability under the ADA. The cases involved in this attempt to clarify the meaning of a disability under the ADA include Sutton v. United Air Lines (527 U.S. 471, June 22, 1999), Murphy v. United Parcel Service Incorporated (527 U.S. 516, June 22, 1999), and Albertsons Incorporated v. Kirkingburg (527 U.S. 555, June 22, 1999) (Pardeck, 2001).

In Sutton v. United Air Lines, identical twin sisters on the basis of poor eyesight were denied pilot positions. Both sisters had 20/20 corrected vision and had considerable experienced as commercial pilots with regional airlines. United Airlines requires pilots to have at least 20/100 vision in each eye without any corrective measures. The sisters' claim they were covered under the ADA since without corrective measures their eyesight is poor enough to substantially limit a major life activity, seeing. The airline countered that because their sight is normal with corrective measures the sisters were not disabled under the ADA. A lower federal court ruled in favor of United Airlines; in the summer of 1999, the Supreme Court upheld this lower court decision (Pardeck, 2001).

Murphy v. United Parcel Service Incorporated involved Vaughn Murphy who was a mechanic with United Parcel Service. Murphy began working for United Parcel in 1994 as a mechanic. As a mechanic, Murphy was required to have a Department of Transportation (DOT) health card because he would need to drive large trucks for road checks. Murphy's initial physical exam cleared him and he was given a DOT health card and commercial driver's license. A month later, a blood pressure reading showed his blood pressure to be above DOT guidelines; he was fired by United Parcel because of his blood pressure level. Murphy claimed he had a disability under the ADA because without medication he could not carry out major life activities. Murphy argued that United Parcel should allow him to adjust his medication in order to lower his blood pressure to a level acceptable to the DOT health guidelines as a reasonable accommodation. A lower court ruled in favor of United Parcel. The court held that Murphy was terminated because his blood pressure exceeded the DOT's requirement and therefore was not a qualified individual with a disability. In 1999 the Supreme Court upheld the lower federal court's ruling (Pardeck, 2001).

The third employment case involved Albertsons Incorporated v. Kirkingburg. In 1990, Kirkingburg, a truck driver, passed the necessary tests for a license despite limited vision in one eye. Kirkingburg was erroneously certified by the Department of Transportation and granted his commercial truck driver license. When Kirkingburg was correctly assessed in 1992, he was told that he had to get a waiver of the DOT standards under a waiver program begun that year. Albertsons, however, fired him for failing to meet the basic DOT vision standards and refused to rehire him after he received a waiver. Kirkingburg filed a discrimination lawsuit under the ADA against Albertsons. A lower federal court ruled that Kirkingburg was not qualified without an accommodation because he could not meet the basic DOT standards and that the waiver program did not alter those standards. An appeals court ruled that Kirkingburg had established a disability under the ADA by demonstrating that the manner in which he sees differed significantly from the regulations in setting a job-related vision standard. Furthermore, Alberston could not use compliance with the DOT regulations to justify its requirement because the waiver program was a legitimate part of the DOT regulatory scheme (Pardeck, 2001).

Albertsons Incorporated v. Kirkingburg was appealed to the United States Supreme Court. The Supreme Court reversed the Appeals Court ruling. The Supreme Court held that an employers' right to set safety guidelines or adhere to federal guidelines was seen as enough reason to refuse to hire or fire an individual. Furthermore, even if the DOT waived the sight guidelines on an experimental basis, employers do not have to waiver their safety standards (Pardeck, 2001).

In Sutton v. United Airlines, Murphy v. United Parcel Service, and Albertsons v. Kirkingburg, the United States Supreme Court ruled against the plaintiffs in all three employment cases. In the Sutton case, the Supreme Court found that whether an individual has a disability as defined by the ADA depends upon the effect of one's condition or impairment "in reference to the measures that mitigate the individual's impairment." In other words, people should be evaluated on the basis of their condition with the use of medication or assistive devices when determining whether their disability substantially limits major life functioning. The same line of reasoning applied to the Murphy v. United Parcel Service and Albertsons v. Kirkingburg (Pardeck, 2001).

Title I

In the Board of Trustees of the University of Alabama v. Garrett (531 U.S. 356, Feb 21, 2001) the question answered was whether the 11th Amendment bars employees of a state from recovering monetary damages from the state for violations of Title I of the ADA. The Court held that Suits by employees of a state to recover money damages from the state for violations of Title I of the ADA are barred by the 11th Amendment. However, in footnote 9 of the opinion, the Court indicated that Title I of the ADA is still applicable to the states, and can be enforced by the United States in actions for money damages. Regardless of this footnote in the opinion, the Court greatly weakened the protections of state employees under Title I of the ADA.

Title II

Olmstead v. L.C. (527 U.S. 581, June 22, 1999) has far reaching effects on disability services provided by state and local government. The plaintiffs in this case were two intellectually and emotionally impaired patients who were institutionalized in the state of Georgia. The plaintiffs claimed that they were denied services in the most integrated setting because they were placed in an institutional care. They claimed that institutionalization segregated them from the rest of society unnecessarily. The doctors for the plaintiffs found that community based treatment was more appropriate for their conditions and treatment needs (Pardeck, 2001).

A lower federal court ruled in favor of the plaintiffs finding that when the state confines an individual in an institutionalized setting when a community placement is more appropriate violates a core principle underlying the ADA, that being to integrate persons with disabilities into the larger society. Olmstead v. L. C. was appealed to the Supreme Court; the Court ruled that the institutionalization of mentally disabled people is a form of discrimination and that the state of Georgia violated the plaintiff's rights under the ADA (Pardeck, 2001).

Tennessee v. Lane is currently being considered by the United States Supreme Court. In 1998, George Lane and Beverly Jones brought a lawsuit against the State of Tennessee under Title II of the ADA alleging that several courthouses in the state were inaccessible to a person who uses a wheelchair. They filed suit under Title II, which prohibits governmental entities from denying public services, programs and activities to individuals on the basis of their disability. In addition, it provides that persons who have been harmed by discrimination can seek damages from governmental entities, including the states. The Lane case raises an extremely important issue: Does Congress have the power to override the states' immunity from suit and authorize Title II plaintiffs to seek damages from the states? If the Court rules in favor of the State of Tennessee, it will mean plaintiffs can no longer seek damages from states. Consequently, Title II will have only a limited impact in protecting those who are discriminated against by states on the basis of disability.

The rulings by the United States Supreme Court over the last 10 years have had a profound impact on the ADA. Even though a number of these rulings have strengthened some aspects of the ADA, others have greatly limited the impact of the ADA. Specifically, the definition of a disability has been narrowed. Title I now only provides limited protec tion for state employees. In Tennessee v. Lane, currently before the Court, a ruling in favor of the State of Tennessee will mean states will no longer have to insure government buildings and programs need to be accessible to persons with disabilities. Much needs to be done in the 21st Century in the area of disability law, particularly the strengthening of the ADA by Congress, to insure that persons with disabilities receive protection from discrimination by public and private entities.

THE EQUAL EMPLOYMENT OPPORTUNITY COMMISSION (EEOC) ENFORCEMENT OF TITLE I

Since the passage of the ADA, the EEOC has taken an active and forceful role in removing barriers and increasing opportunities for people with disabilities in the workplace. Nearly a quarter of the EEOC's caseload is comprised of discrimination complaints under Title I of the ADA. The EEOC has taken a number of ADA employment cases to court; the agency prevailed in nearly 90 percent of these cases. There have been 126,000 charges of discrimination under Title I; 15 percent have been resolved in favor of the individual. Since the enactment of the ADA, $261 million in payments and other benefits have been won by the EEOC for persons with disabilities in the workplace. Keep in mind that prior to the enactment of the ADA, a person with a disability could be terminated from a job because of a disability. Such behavior by an employer is now illegal under the ADA (Castro, 2000).

Numerous individuals with disabilities have received monetary and non-monetary benefits through the enforcement efforts of the EEOC. The following are examples of some of the cases that were settled by the EEOC without using litigation (Castro, 2000).

- A large drug store chain, which receives over 50,000 applications yearly, changed its job application form by removing unlawful pre-employment inquiries about applicants' disabilities.
- A defense contractor agreed to change its policy requiring employees to disclose their use of prescription medication on an ongoing basis.
- A state law requiring a GED or high school diploma for day care positions was changed to recognize "Certificate of Learning" granted to individuals with intellectual disabilities.
- A person with diabetes was denied a position as a firefighter based on the employer's generalized assessment that his condition would prevent him from safely performing his job. The evidence collected by the EEOC concluded that the individual had safely performed as a volunteer firefighter for 11 years and that his medical condition posed no threat for a firefighter position. The employer hired the person and provided monetary relief.
- A person with disfigurement of her face and head was denied a job at a bookstore, even though she was qualified for the job. The employer was concerned about customers' reactions to her appearance. The employer agreed to give her the job and provided monetary relief.

The EEOC has filed 416 lawsuits on behalf of persons with disabilities. The following summarizes some of these important lawsuits (Castro, 2000).

- The very first lawsuit filed by the EEOC under the ADA was the EEOC and Charles Wessel v. AIC Security Investigation, Ltd. Charles Wessel was fired from his position because he had terminal brain cancer. The jury ruled in favor of Wessel; he was awarded $22,000 in back pay, $50,000 in compensatory damages, and $150,000 in punitive damages.
- The Commission in EEOC v. Professional Nurses, Inc. won a verdict in favor of a highly qualified nurse who was denied employment because of her history of schizophrenia.

- In the EEOC v. Union Carbide, the Commission sued Union Carbide when it refused to provide a reasonable accommodation for an employee with a bipolar disorder. The employee requested that he be assigned to a non-rotating shift schedule; the company fired him because of his request and disability. He was awarded $120,000 in compensatory damages and Union Carbide agreed to provide accommodations for employees with disabilities in the future.
- In the EEOC v. Showbiz Pizza Time Inc., a jury found that a custodian with mental retardation was fired because of his disability. A manager stated he did not want his company to employ "those type of people." The jury awarded the fired employee $70,000 in compensatory damages for emotional distress and 13 million in punitive damages which were later reduced. The judge ordered back pay and the reinstatement of the employee.
- In EEOC v. The Kroger Company, a favorable verdict resulted for a cashier with paraplegia who could not use the store's rest room or break room because they were located down a flight of stairs. The company agreed to build an accessible bathroom and break room. The company also provided the employee with $225,000 in compensatory and punitive damages.
- In EEOC v. El Chico Restaurants of Louisiana, Inc., the Commission challenged a restaurant's refusal to hire a job applicant as a dishwasher because he was blind. During the job interview the applicant was not even allowed to demonstrate how he could do the job. The restaurant agreed to provide the applicant with $24,000 in monetary relief and to provide training for all its managers on issues related to the ADA.
- The Commission claimed in EEOC v. Guardmark that a security guard was fired because he had insulin-dependent diabetes. The company reimbursed the guard $25,000 in back pay and compensatory damages and donated $25,000 to a scholarship fund for persons with disabilities.
- In EEOC v. Armstrong Brothers Tool Company, the Commission challenged the company's firing of a sales representative because he had epilepsy and previously had surgery for a brain tumor. The company agreed to pay the former employee $27,000 in back pay and $108,000 in compensatory damages.

ADVOCACY
AND THE AMERICANS WITH DISABILITIES ACT

The Americans With Disabilities Act is clearly grounded in the human rights perspective. The ADA, like other civil rights legislation of the past, is aimed at an oppressed group, persons with disabilities, who have been denied equal opportunity to participate in American society (Pardeck, 1998).

It is important to note that under the ADA, persons with disabilities are viewed as a minority group. This perspective suggests, for example, that if a person with a disability is poor, it is less a result of a personal inadequacy than of a discriminatory society (Federal Register, 1980). Consequently, the adjustment to a disability is not merely a personal trouble but one that requires the larger society to change its views concerning persons with disabilities (Fiedler, 1978). In other words, society must change its attitudes and stereotypes; it must also remove the obstacles it has placed in the way of self-fulfillment for people with disabilities, including inaccessible transportation and architectural systems designed only for the able (Karger & Stoesz, 1994).

Like other oppressed groups within American society, people with disabilities have suffered tremendous discrimination (Ianacone, 1977). The National Council on Disability, the Civil Rights Commission, and national polls all conclude that discrimination against people with disabilities is pervasive in American society (Pardeck & Chung, 1992). This discrimination is sometimes in the form of prejudice, patronizing attitudes, and still at other times it is the result of indifference (Burgdorf & Burgdorf, 1977). Regardless of the origin, the outcomes are the same: exclusion, segregation, or the denial of equal, effective, and meaningful opportunities to participate in activities and programs (Brothwell & Sandison, 1967). The goal of the ADA is preventing and correcting the numerous problems associated with discrimination against people with disabilities (Pardeck & Chung, 1992). A basic social work strategy, advocacy, can be effective as a means for ensuring the ADA is implemented appropriately (Pardeck, 1998).

The goals of advocacy are to achieve social justice and to empower people. Advocacy helps people correct those situations that are unjust. Achieving social justice through advocacy requires the active participation of citizens who are vulnerable or disenfranchised; the professional social worker also plays a critical role in this process. The banding together of those who wish to achieve social justice provides the opportunity for empowerment, for active, responsible participation in the public realm (Lewis, 1992). The role of the advocate is to speak on behalf of clients and to empower clients to speak on their own behalf in situations where their rights have been denied. The advocacy role is a critical strategy for those who are grounded in a social justice approach to practice because it expands opportunities by protecting the interests of clients. Furthermore, advocacy is a classic role aimed at changing the oppressive social environments of clients, including the various systems that prevent individual growth and development (Pardeck, 1998).

McGowan (1987) concludes that advocacy can be conducted at two levels, case advocacy and cause advocacy. The case advocacy approach focuses on individual cases. It involves the partisan intervention on behalf of a client or identified client group with one or more secondary institutions to secure or enhance needed services, resources, or entitlements (McGowan, 1987). Cause advocacy seeks to redress collective issues through social change efforts and improving social policies (Pardeck, 1998).

Rees (1991) argues that case and cause advocacy both begin by identifying the dynamics causing social injustice. Rees makes the following conclusion about the advocacy process:

> The decision to pursue the advocacy of a case or a cause, or a combination of both, will usually have been preceded by the identification of an injustice which it is felt cannot be rectified simply by efficient administration or negotiation. The identification of an injustice and the sense of conviction concerning the removal of this injustice should become a priority. . . It is not sufficient merely to recognize an injustice. You have to believe that this issue should be fought for and if necessary over a long period of time. The effective advocacy role involves data collection, effective communication with the public through the media, raising revenues, and building coalitions. (p. 146)

Miley, O'Melia, and DuBois (1995) conclude that the following issues must be an integral part of the advocacy process aimed at social injustice and social change:

1. The location of the problem must be identified. It must be determined, for example, whether the problem reflects a personal need, a gap in services, or inequitable social policy.

2. The objectives of intervention must be identified. For instance, objectives might be defined as procuring entitlements for clients or expanding job opportunities for oppressed individuals.
3. The target system of advocacy intervention must be identified. This at times might be the practitioner's own agency or other systems the agency works with.
4. The advocate must determine what authority or sanction he or she has to intervene in a targeted system. This can include legal rights of clients and judicial decisions.
5. The resources available for advocacy efforts must be identified. These resources include professional expertise, political influence, and one's credibility and reputation.
6. It must be determined by those involved in an advocacy effort the degree to which the target system is receptive to the proposed advocacy effort. The target system will make this decision based on the reasonableness or lawfulness of the advocacy effort.
7. The level at which the intervention will occur must be analyzed to insure that the desired outcomes will be achieved. Different levels of intervention might include policy changes, modification of administrative procedures, and alterations in the discretionary actions taken by staff or management in an agency.
8. The object of intervention must be identified. This might include individual delivery services, agency administrators, or even a legislative body.
9. The strategies of advocacy intervention must be determined. These strategies include the roles of negotiator, collaborator, and adversary.
10. Those involved in advocacy efforts must learn from the outcomes of prior advocacy efforts, including both failures and successes.

What should be clear from the above information is the degree to which it is consistent with a social justice approach to practice. Furthermore, the above points suggest that advocacy is a holistic approach to social change that involves efforts at both the micro and macro levels (Pardeck, 1998).

Those who are involved in advocacy efforts must understand the need for this type of intervention with the various systems they work with (Pardeck, 1998). What must be understood, if one considers the plight of people with disabilities, is that public and private entities did not, for example, ask for the passage of the Americans With Disabilities

Act. Most systems located in the public and private sectors, including schools and businesses, would prefer self-regulation over a federal mandate aimed at protecting people with disabilities. Those involved in advocacy find that self-regulation does not work and that even after the passage of legislation such as the Americans With Disabilities Act, social systems mandated to conform to this new disability law will attempt to avoid their legal obligations. This means advocacy is an absolute necessity to insure laws, such as the Americans With Disabilities Act, are implemented appropriately (Pardeck, 1998).

There are a number of reasons why entities legally bound by the mandates of civil rights legislation such as the ADA attempt to avoid compliance. First, organizations including schools and private businesses have been provided the compliance materials for the Americans With Disabilities Act; however, they often do not follow procedures set forth in compliance materials because they may contradict the bureaucratic rules of these systems. For example, the person with a disability brings a unique set of needs to the workplace, including the need at times for reasonable accommodations. Bureaucratic organizations are often rigid systems and are not prone to make exceptions; they literally must be forced to make exceptions through strong advocacy efforts (Pardeck, 1998).

Second, all public and private entities bound by the mandates of the ADA feel that they operate on limited resources. If an employee with a disability requests a reasonable accommodation in order to do his or her job, the organization understands this to be an added cost. Advocates must play the role of convincing organizations asked to provide special accommodations for people with disabilities that this is a requirement of the law, and that the federal mandate for providing reasonable accommodations is based on the needs of the person with a disability and not necessarily on the needs of the organization's budget (Pardeck, 1998).

Third, often people are intimidated by both public and private bureaucracies. For example, a person with a disability may have limited experience and exposure in dealing with organizations in general. Such persons need the help of an expert, the advocate, in dealing with complex organizations. Skillful advocates understand how complex organizations work and are well aware of the regulations these systems must follow, including disability laws (Pardeck, 1998).

Lastly, often it is difficult for persons with disabilities to look at their own problems without their emotions impacting their objectivity. Skillful advocates are able to step back from situations that negatively impact persons with disabilities and provide reason and objectivity to the process for both the person with a disability and the entity who is not complying with the ADA (Pardeck, 1998).

With the ADA as an example, the importance of advocacy even after a law has been passed to protect a category of people becomes clear. Advocacy is about influence and power, ingredients that are often critical to forcing entities to conform to regulations and laws (Pardeck, 1998).

Effective Advocacy Skills for Persons with Disabilities

The ADA and other disability laws were enacted to protect the rights of people with disabilities; the history of the ADA suggests that persons with disabilities played a critical role in the creation of this law (Pardeck and Chung, 1991). People with disabilities have a primary responsibility for ensuring that their rights are met under the mandates of the ADA. This can only be achieved if persons with disabilities learn how to effectively advocate on their own behalf. The following strategies and skills are designed to help persons with disabilities become effective advocates for themselves. The goals of the following are to empower persons with disabilities to achieve social justice for themselves and others with disabilities (Pardeck, 1998).

Believing in Their Rights

Persons with disabilities must be taught that they are equal partners with others, such as professional social workers, who are involved with advocacy efforts. Equal partnership also means that a person with a disability must accept his or her share of responsibility for solving problems related to advocacy efforts.

Having a Clear Vision

Persons with disabilities must learn to communicate clearly with systems that are denying them their rights under the ADA. They must be optimistic about what can be achieved as a result of advocacy. While trying to achieve what is perceived as ideal, they must be able to recognize what is realistic.

Organization

Persons with disabilities must be taught to understand that being organized is an absolute necessity to effective advocacy. They must know how to file information, keep track of records, and organize important documentation critical to the advocacy process. The person with a disability should be encouraged to date all materials and to make duplicate copies of all documents.

Prioritizing

Persons with disabilities must develop skills in learning how to decide what the most important issues are related to their advocacy efforts. This should be based on their greatest needs as a person with a disability. One useful technique for prioritizing needs is to write them down on paper and then prioritize them in order of importance.

Understanding One's Disabilities

A person with a disability must learn everything possible about his or her disability. It is important to acquire in-depth information about one's own medical needs, as well as the various assistive technology available to one as possible reasonable accommodations in the workplace or other settings. In general, persons with disabilities often know more than professionals about their own special needs. It is important for a person with a disability to share information about his or her disability with the entity that is denying that person legal rights under the ADA. This information may help in the resolution of the problem between the person with a disability and an unresponsive system.

Knowing the Law

Persons with disabilities must learn about their rights under the ADA. They also should become familiar with their rights under other federal disability laws. By knowing these laws, they will be better able to advocate for their rights.

Following the Chain of Command

It is important for a person with a disability to know that effective advocacy means he or she should first engage those persons that can correct a problem at the lower levels of an organization. These individuals should be allowed the opportunity to address issues before the person with a disability moves to higher levels of organizations. If results cannot be obtained at a lower level, then the individual with a disability must move systematically up the chain of command.

Being Informative

The person with a disability must understand his or her special needs. He or she should be able to convey all relevant information about his or her disability to the system that advocacy efforts are aimed at. This strategy can be helpful in resolving the problem between the person with a disability and the system denying the person's rights under the ADA.

Offering Solutions

The person with a disability needs to be creative in finding solutions to problems that call for advocacy efforts. Positive solutions are those that benefit everyone involved in the advocacy process. This kind of strategy can mean a successful resolution to the advocacy process.

Being Principled and Persistent

It is important for a person with a disability to master the art of being clear to officials about needed changes; one must be firm on these changes. It is important to keep at the advocacy process and not to let the battle become the issue. The person with a disability must avoid being adversarial and realize that he or she must be assertive and not aggressive. One must have a vision that the issue will be resolved to his or her satisfaction. It is best to assume that the system one is aiming advocacy efforts toward has honorable intentions.

Learning to Communicate Effectively

A person with a disability must understand that many problems result from poor communication between parties. It is important to learn to listen to what others are saying and to realize that others may have valuable insights into a confronting problem. If a person with a disability does not understand something, he or she must ask questions. It is important to be sincere and honest, and say what is really meant. Effective communication involves smiling and being relaxed, and not making others defensive. It is a good idea for a person with a disability to follow up conversations and meetings with a written summary of the discussion and agreements made.

Letting Others Know When Pleased

It is important to let the system that has changed because of advocacy efforts hear the person's satisfaction and excitement as the system continues to progress in the area of ADA rights. This kind of positive behavior will help to keep the organization on the right track in the area of disability law.

Developing Endurance

One of the first lessons learned from doing advocacy is that it is important to learn to develop endurance. Advocacy is a process that often extends over a long time period. The person with a disability will face many challenges and issues; some successes and some failures need to be expected. It is important to learn lessons from both. The person with a disability must realize that if he or she has been successful in advocacy, for example, with an employer, that his or her relationship is likely to be long term with that employer. Effective advocacy skills will help make this relationship a positive one.

Following Through

One must make a concerted effort to monitor the process concerning what has been agreed to as a result of the advocacy process. The person with a disability must make sure the accommodation or program changes are being provided appropriately. If the need for a different accommodation emerges, it is critical to advocate for these changes.

Having a Sense of Humor

Advocacy is about endurance. Developing and cultivating a sense of humor is one of the most important traits a person with a disability needs for successful advocacy.

CONCLUSIONS

In this paper, the author has overviewed the key components of the ADA. A discussion was offered on why and how persons with disabilities are discriminated against. The standard stereotypes often heard about persons with disabilities were offered. Critical United States Supreme Court decisions were presented; many of these decisions have greatly limited the power of the ADA in protecting the rights of persons with disabilities. Even though the United States Supreme Court has narrowed the impact of the ADA in American life, a number of EEOC cases were presented in the paper which suggests this Federal agency is attempting to protect persons with disabilities against discrimination. The final area covered in the paper dealt with the topic of advocacy; advocacy may well be one of the most effective tools to help insure that the rights of people with disabilities are protected.

Clearly, in the 21st century, the ADA is the most important civil rights law for persons with disabilities. Even though many of the initial intentions of the ADA have been negated by the United States Supreme Court, countless people with disabilities have benefitted from the protections of the ADA. What is critical at this time is the United States Congress must pass legislation that corrects the attacks on the ADA by the Court. Persons with disabilities need to be advocates for these changes in the legislative process.

REFERENCES

Americans With Disabilities Act of 1990 (The). (1990). P. L. 101-336, 105 Stat. 327, 42 U.S.C., 12101 et seq.

Arnold, K. (1999). Americans With Disabilities Act: Do cancer patients qualify as disabled? *Journal of the National Cancer Institute*, 91, 822-825.

Brothwell, D. S., & Sandison, A. T. (1967). *Diseases in antiquity.* Springfield, IL: Charles C. Thomas.

Burgdorf, R. L., & Burgdorf, M. P. (1977). The wicked witch is almost dead: Buck v. Bell and the sterilization of handicapped persons. *Temple Law Quarterly*, 50, 995-1054.

Castro, I. L. (2000). *A report on the tenth anniversary of the Americans With Disabilities Act (ADA).* http://www.eeoc.gov/ada/statusreport.html

Equal Employment Opportunity Commission & U. S. Department of Justice (1992). The Americans With Disabilities Act: Questions and answers. Washington, DC: National Institute on Disabilities and Rehabilitation Research.

Federal Register (1980). No. 66. Washington, DC: U. S. Printing.

Harrison, M., & Gilbert, S. (Eds) (1992). *The Americans With Disabilities Act handbook.* Beverly Hills, CA: Excellent Books.

Hugo, V. (1991). *Hunchback of Notre Dame.* New York: Bantam Doubleday.

Karger, H. J., & Stoesz, D. (1994). *American Social Welfare: A Pluralist Approach* (2nd ed). White Plains, NY: Longman.

Lewis, E. (1992). Social change and citizen action: A philosophical exploration for modern social group work. *Social work with Groups*, 14, 23-34.

Livenel, H. (1982). On the origins of negative attitudes toward people with disabilities. *Rehabilitation Literature*, 43, 280-283.

Longmore, P. K. (1987). Uncovering the hidden history of people with disabilities. *Reviews in American History*, 15, 355-364.

Mackelprang, R., & Salsgiver, R. (1999). *Disability: A diversity model approach in human service practice.* Pacific Grove, CA: Brooks/Cole Publishing Company.

McGowan, B. G. (1987). Advocacy. In A. Minahan (Ed.), *Encyclopedia of social work: Vol. 1* (18th ed., pp. 89-95). Silver Spring, MD: National Association of Social Workers.

Miley, K. K., O'Melia, M., & DuBois, B. (1995). *Generalist social work practice: An empowering approach.* Boston: Allyn and Bacon.

Pardeck, J. T. (2002). Knowledge, Tasks and Strategies for Teaching about Persons with Disabilities: Implications for Social Work Education. *Journal of Social Work in Disability & Rehabilitation*, 1, 53-72.

Pardeck, J. T. (1998). *Social Work after the Americans With Disabilities Act: New Challenges and Opportunities for Social Service Professionals.* Westport, CT: Auburn House.

Pardeck, J. T. (2001). An update on the Americans With Disabilities Act: Implications for health and human services delivery. *Journal of Health & Social Policy*, 13, 1-15.

Pardeck, J. T., & Chung, W. (1992). An analysis of the Americans With Disabilities Act of 1990. *Journal of Health & Social Policy*, 4, 47-56.

Rees, S. (1991). *Achieving power: Practice and policy in social welfare.* North Sydney, Australia: Allen & Unwin.

SECTION III
DISABILITY THEORY
IN THE TWENTY-FIRST CENTURY

Social Norms and Their Implications
for Disability

John W. Murphy

SUMMARY. This paper discusses how and why the norms for defining disability continue to change. This analysis illustrates the social nature of the disability and that changing norms continue to define the meaning of disability. The paper is grounded in a postmodern perspective, a notion that has only entered the field of disability in the 21st century. *[Article copies available for a fee from The Haworth Document Delivery Service: 1-800-HAWORTH. E-mail address: <docdelivery@haworthpress.com> Website: <http://www.HaworthPress.com> © 2005 by The Haworth Press, Inc. All rights reserved.]*

John W. Murphy, PhD, is Professor of Sociology, University of Miami, Department of Sociology, 5202 University Drive, Merrick Building, Room 120, Coral Gables, FL 33124-2035.

[Haworth co-indexing entry note]: "Social Norms and Their Implications for Disability." Murphy, John W. Co-published simultaneously in *Journal of Social Work in Disability & Rehabilitation* (The Haworth Social Work Practice Press, an imprint of The Haworth Press, Inc.) Vol. 4, No. 1/2, 2005, pp. 153-163; and: *Disability Issues for Social Workers and Human Services Professionals in the Twenty-First Century* (ed: John W. Murphy, and John T. Pardeck) The Haworth Social Work Practice Press, an imprint of The Haworth Press, Inc., 2005, pp. 153-163. Single or multiple copies of this article are available for a fee from The Haworth Document Delivery Service [1-800-HAWORTH, 9:00 a.m. - 5:00 p.m. (EST). E-mail address: docdelivery@haworthpress.com].

KEYWORDS. Postmodernism, disability, norms, social construct, theory, culture

Disability does not stand alone, but exists within a normative context. Nonetheless, this declaration does not necessarily clarify matters. Simply referring to the social background of norms, accordingly, does not automatically provide much insight into the nature of disability or any other trait. Stated differently, norms are accompanied by a conceptual framework that must be clarified, before any social phenomenon can be properly understood. In other words, norms have a history and assume various forms that are not predetermined.

The point is not simply that norms change, but their fundamental status has been altered over time. Philosophers refer to this basic nature as their ontological character. During the late nineteenth century, for example, norms were thought to epitomize reason and were treated as universal. In the early twentieth century, however, this viewpoint was challenged by those who thought that the mind and rules of normativeness are inextricably linked. Norms were thus accepted to be embedded within layers of cultural praxis and were no longer treated as obtrusive. Soon norms were portrayed as symbolic or constructed, and thus labeling specific persons as inherently unacceptable became inappropriate.

But despite this change in attitude, pluralism has not been achieved. Disabled persons face discrimination, although they are described in more holistic terms. Instead of a hostile world, they are described as encountering challenges. The problem is that norms have not yet been addressed in a manner required to produce true pluralism. Discrimination is still experienced by people with disabilities, but in much more sophisticated ways than in the past. Rather than barring people with disabilities from certain jobs, they are simply portrayed as fulfilling their unique potential by occupying very different social roles. The so-called essential qualities of persons with disabilities are recognized as the reason why they should be treated differently.

But due to recent changes in sociological theory, norms no longer have to be universal to secure social order. Pluralism, therefore, is not simply a utopian ideal promoted by dreamers. Nonetheless, more work needs to be done to insure that all persons are integrated into society without violating how they define themselves. Specifically, failure to assimilate to a specific normative referent should not condemn persons such as those with disabilities to the margins of society. Likewise, cultural and other modes of diversity, such as a disability, no longer have to be viewed as a threat to social integrity.

CLASSIC THEORY AND MORAL ORDER

The origin of modern sociological theory is usually thought to be Nineteenth Century France. Both Comte and Durkheim were living in a society they thought was on the brink of chaos (Aron, 1968, pp. 83-92). Rapid industrialization was introducing values that stressed individualism, social mobility, and the accumulation of material wealth. As a result, tradition was devalued, along with community solidarity. And given these conditions, these authors feared that French society was in the midst of a spiritual breakdown. There was nothing available, in other words, to bind persons together into a lasting moral order.

If French society was going to continue, a new normative base would be needed. This foundation would have to be powerful enough, however, to counteract the new image of the citizen that was emerging—an autonomous person who has few social ties and obligations. Norms, accordingly, would have to be substantial enough to withstand demands for increased freedom and personal responsibility, or social fragmentation would continue unabated.

Comte and Durkheim, therefore, argued that norms should be treated as objective and thus universal. But to achieve this status, these rules would have to be linked to science. Such an association was not necessarily rare at the time. After all, science was presumed to be value-free and capable of generating knowledge in an unbiased manner. Therefore, the resulting information would not be limited by perspective and have universal appeal. Any rational person, in this regard, would appreciate these norms because of their scientific origin and unrestricted applicability.

This theoretical maneuver inaugurated a trend in viewing social order that continues today. Valid norms, simply put, transcend cultural contingencies and are considered immune to interpretation or critique. To keep society together, borrowing from (Durkheim 1983, p. 101) norms are presumed to exist sui generis. All persons have to do to preserve order is to assimilate and internalize these universal standards.

In the end, the key message is that society cannot survive without this sort of uniformity. This point was reinforced by Talcott Parsons (1963, pp. 36-45), and his brand of functionalism, when he described social order to be a structural system that is unified by stable and universal values. In the absence of this homogeneity, he envisioned the Hobbesian debacle to be inevitable. According to this theory, persons could not be trusted to work together and achieve even a minimal consensus without appreciable coercion.

Norms, therefore, had to be viewed as categorically removed from the citizenry, or these regulations would not have the stature necessary to prevail for very long. Behavioral expectations, for example, could be tainted by personal preferences and considered optional, unless standards are autonomous and beyond reproach. In view of this treatment of norms, there should be no wonder why diversity has become anathema to the maintenance of order. Nowadays even a very limited pluralism has come to represent a failure to assimilate and an affront to rationality. Without a strong commitment to a single language, culture, and history most persons believe that a nation is doomed.

All persons, accordingly, are expected to function in a relatively similar manner. Exceptions are possible, but these individuals must have very good excuses for their inability to adapt. But at no time should they be allowed to challenge or alter the norm; they should simply be tolerated and happy with their marginal position in society. Consistent with the functionalist position, they should be granted specific roles that enable them to survive on the periphery of the mainstream.

THE LINGUISTIC TURN

During the 1960s, a change in theory occurred that Durkheim (1983) announced years earlier would be disastrous to modern societies. Specifically, the dualism that enabled norms to be approached as if they were autonomous was undermined. A point Durkheim thought was very problematic with respect to pragmatism became reality–that is, the mind and reality were encouraged to mingle too closely. As a consequence of the so-called linguistic turn, knowledge was declared to be mediated completely by speech acts that could never be overcome.

Influenced by G.H. Mead, symbolic interactionists such as Herbert Blumer (1969) announced that reality is symbolic rather than objective. In this case, language does not merely highlight events but is imagined to be a creative force. And as a result of changes in definition, now understood as the application of labels, the nature of reality can be dramatically transformed. Accordingly, the objective base of morality sought by Comte and Durkheim is in jeopardy, for norms are now mired in subjectivity.

Continuing this trend, but under the sway of phenomenology, ethno-methodologists argued that facts are not things–the hallmark of Durk-heim's stance on norms–but accomplishments (Garfinkel, 1967). Because phenomenologists claim consciousness is always conscious of something, facts are acknowledged to be constructed consciously and maintained through continued interaction between persons. Facts, in other words, are a product of intentionality, and thus norms are not objective but revealed through on-going discourse. Those that become prominent are elevated in importance because of shifts in values, beliefs, or commitments.

Due to this tie between consciousness and reality, the social world is referred to by phenomenologists and ethnomethodologists as the *Lebenswelt*, or life-world. By using this language they are suggesting that the world is not simply empirical but alive with meaning and significance. The social world has a living texture that is maintained through interaction and a commitment to particular norms. These prejudices, furthermore, determine how persons respond to events and the comportment of others.

By the arrival of the 1990s, this approach had assumed a decidedly political cast (Choi and Murphy, 1992, pp. 61-64). Advocates of multiculturalism, that includes persons with disabilities, for example, argued that not only are norms–along with fact and truth–a product of interests, political power plays a large role in specifying which standards are considered normal and generally acceptable. As some critics such as Stanley Fish (1989, p. 251) maintained, truth has always been thoroughly politicized, although realists in the Durkheimian mold chose to overlook this connection.

Multiculturalists charged that language use is central to organizing reality, and therefore norms are thoroughly interpretive. This means that language plays a critical role in defining disability and its meaning. Reminiscent of the later Wittgenstein, establishing norms is described to be a game (Lyotard, 1983, pp. 9-11). And as a result of the linguistic maneuvers that are made, some norms become more relevant than others. Personal traits or actions, accordingly, no longer have inherent meaning or value. Depending on the language game in use, and the labels that are invoked, a person's identity can be defined in any number of ways.

Some critics found this view of norms to be very liberating. Because norms are never automatically universal, but gain validity only through individual or collective assent, identities can be (re)constructed almost interminably. Rather than an objective feature of action, a disability is conceptualized in a cultural context. Multiculturalists, accordingly, claim that social life is much more complex and variegated than writers such as Durkheim or Parsons could tolerate.

The central shortcoming of this rejection of dualism is that subjectivity is merely juxtaposed to objectivity. Hence subjective judgments can be treated as simply opinions that have little to do with the real state of affairs. A person may feel adequate, for example, but the actual quality of his or her performance cannot be ignored. And if persons continue to be confused about this difference, they may eventually lose all credibility. Various writers, accordingly, began to think seriously about how human praxis could be given more validity.

GOING BEYOND SUBJECTIVITY

During the late 1990s a new and quite radical social philosophy arrived on the intellectual scene. This viewpoint is called quantum aesthetics, and was associated originally with a group of artists and writers in Grenada, Spain. Gregorio Morales (1998), a writer, is the intellectual leader of this group, which now includes participants from throughout the world.

Although he was influenced by postmodernism, particularly the emphasis that was placed on language games, Morales gradually became disenchanted with this philosophical movement. His principal concern was that this linguistic theory did not alter appreciably the traditional conception of reality. In his opinion, language was treated as simply another facet of reality, albeit one that is granted increasing importance. Nonetheless, language could not subvert the demands issued by traditional social institutions, for example, because speech is still basically subjective and incapable of altering objectivity.

Proponents of quantum aesthetics, accordingly, took their inspiration from the "uncertainty principle" of Heisenberg (Caro and Murphy, 2003). What he noticed is that the structure of an experiment determines the identity of the phenomenon that is studied. For example, in one situation light behaves like a wave and in another a particle. Light, in other words, can be both a wave and a particle, depending on how an experiment is organized. This discovery led him to declare that researchers tend to find what they set out to investigate.

Given this fluctuation, Heisenberg concluded that reality is not very stable, and that the human presence has a lot to do with the fundamental nature of the world. As quantum physicists are fond of saying, the act of measurement collapses the wave function in one way or another, thereby defining reality. If something as primordial as light can be manipulated in this manner, Heisenberg surmised that reality is neither autonomous nor objective. Human intervention was thus understood to extend to the core of reality, wherever this place may be located. In fact, Jean Gebser (1985, p. 544) characterized this demise of objectivity by proclaiming that such a center is elusive and may be established anywhere.

The implications of this theoretical gambit for social existence are obvious. Not only are norms the result of human intervention, but there is no ultimate justification for accepting one rendition over another. Human will, in this sense, is joined inextricably to the fate of persons and their respective perspectives on reality. What must be noted, however, is that this tactic does not necessarily culminate in relativism, as some critics of quantum aesthetics contend.

Within each normative realm that accompanies a specific intervention, certain norms exist that cannot be wantonly abridged. Nonetheless, there is no final rational for any intervention that might be selected and implemented. Although norms exist in each interpretive region of reality, their dominance is secured through the choices that persons make and nothing else. These decisions, however, are not always made in conditions that persons desire, due to the presence of social inequalities or discrimination.

What is presupposed by this thesis is that reality is not something uniform that extends to infinity, but consists of a myriad of normative centers. Each one, additionally, has integrity and should not be violated by any other. In other words, a normative sphere should be extended no farther than the limits prescribed by a particular intervention; norms, accordingly, should not be expanded beyond the parameters imposed by certain epistemological assumptions. As a result, there is nothing especially real about reality, other than the repercussions of making specific choices about the identity of events or behavior.

The contemporary French philosopher Pierre Bourdieu (1992, pp. 120-121) took this outlook seriously and popularized the use of the term *habitus* to describe normative spheres. As he views them, norms are neither subjective nor objective, but reflect commitments that can be publicly verified. His point is that rather than idiosyncratic or universal, norms have an interpretive character that persons have agreed not to question. At least they have been convinced that such questioning would be unproductive. A particular version of normativeness, accordingly, achieves a semblance of stability and can be treated as representing the common weal. Yet in the end, norms are never more than habitual ways of trying to regulate interaction.

SYMBOLIC VIOLENCE

The collapse of dualism inaugurated by quantum aesthetics, along with postmodern critiques, is thought by many writers to have brought many societies to a crucial impasse. Without a cosmopolitan vision, norms begin to proliferate and anomie replaces solidarity. Respect for cultural diversity, which includes persons with disabilities, for example, is believed by many persons to lead inexorably to a loss of social cohesion. In this regard, granting unique rights to various so-called interest groups has culminated in what Schlesinger (1993) calls the "disuniting of America."

As a way of counteracting the accompanying social balkanization, novel attempts have been underway to reestablish fundamental values that all reasonable persons can embrace. And similar to earlier attempts to impose order, these more modern methods must also create the illusion that some norms are undoubtedly universal. Certain norms and values, accordingly, have to be treated as if they are a part of human nature. This kind of treatment is extended to persons with disabilities.

Over the last decade or so, various attempts have been made to distance norms from cultural and other contingencies. Discussions have been initiated, mostly by conservatives, about inherent intelligence, basic social mores, proper languages, and cultural imperatives. The goal of these initiatives is to reestablish normalcy by identifying neutral principles for securing order. A comprehensive foundation is thus available to curb the excesses of multiculturalists and the plethora of liberation movements that have emerged.

These new proponents of social control, however, cannot appear to be as ideological as their adversaries. Their image of appropriate norms or values cannot seem to be politically motivated, or demands for special recognition will continue. Why should conservative values be given special attention, while other positions are dismissed or ignored? As a result, they have engaged in what Bourdieu (1993, pp. 74-81) calls symbolic violence. What they have done, simply stated, is to associate their agenda with allegedly neutral principles, thereby obscuring the political intent of their arguments. The enforcement of constitutional provisions, for example, is described to be predicated on original intent–basic wisdom or rationality–rather than fleeting trends or attempts to protect social entitlements.

In the end, a very sophisticated means of manipulation has been enacted. As a result of severing norms from politics, many citizens have been convinced that these rules are not ideological. Being against civil rights for persons with disabilities, therefore, is portrayed as purely reasonable or logical rather than a political stance that could be interpreted as ableism. Ableism is defined as discrimination based on disability. Those who claim discrimination at the marketplace or their jobs, moreover, are labeled as unprincipled and a threat to the common good. They are complainers who cannot deal with their failures and place their desires above those of society. Persons with disabilities are often viewed as complainers who cannot deal with the problems related to their disabilities.

Assumed by this entire process is the existence of a neutral arbiter of norms. Whereas Durkheim's call for the institution of a reality sui generis was a tour de force, these arguments about basic morals or the utility of competition are more substantial and alluring. They are based on factors such as reason and human nature rather than simply the desire to preserve a particular way of life. Many persons thus engage regularly in their own suppression, because they do not what to violate these cter nal principles. The guilt they would have to endure for transgressing human nature, for example, is too great for them to engage in any protest against their mistreatment. What has been identified as the natural course of events is merely followed.

CONCLUSION: IMPLICATIONS FOR DISABILITY

The introduction of this symbolic mode of social control, however, is not the end of this story. There are numerous critics throughout the world who continue to struggle for an honest pluralism, so that a host of personal and collective identities can flourish. These persons have been influenced by writers, such as Foucault, Bourdieu, and the Frankfurt authors, who realize that a sophisticated epistemological critique is needed to understand the defining and meaning of disability.

These movements operate under the general heading of action "from below" (Murphy and Caro, 2002). What they try to do is (1) illustrate the historical origin of the characteristics that are touted to be a part of the person with a disability, and (2) unravel the process that created these characteristics. The idea is to reveal that there are no universals, other than those that are socially manufactured through education, propaganda, or the exercise of power. Politics is thus shown to be central to the standards or moral foundations that are declared to be neutral. The disability rights movement has been well aware of the politics that defined the inferior status of persons with disabilities.

Hence the question is raised, why should specific persons be inferiorized for political advantage? The point is that in a democracy such marginalization should in general be unacceptable. On the other hand, a disability should be viewed as enriching society. In addition to enhancing the moral quality of a community, a disability should be viewed as contributing to the diversity of the community. How can a society not be enhanced by such a view?

As a result of persons protecting and encouraging one another, a true sense of community might be established. And if no one is treated as an outsider, there are no persons to exploit or degrade. Indeed, those who are part of a community do not tolerate such behavior from other members. Consequently people with disabilities would be fully integrated into society because they are valued for their differences.

Contrary to what Durkheim or Parsons taught, diversity is not automatically anathema to community. Tolerance of a range of norms does not necessarily culminate in anarchy. Through dialogue and the recognition of difference, instead, persons can be integrated into a group without assimilation. But because of the position on order promoted by the mainstream of sociology, this kind of approach to disability is often dismissed as utopian. Most persons are reluctant to accept that cultural or other differences are not inherently a threat to order.

How these differences are handled, in fact, may be the crucial issue, particularly in a democracy. If persons with disabilities are mistreated, for example, they may respond in a manner that suggests their inclusion is unacceptable. However, under other conditions, where no one is threatened, increased diversity may be more satisfying for everyone. One thing is for certain, however; diversity is not declining, and thus new ways must be invented to address this change that are more sensitive than those that have already been tried. And how persons with disabilities are integrated into various cultures may be a true test of democratic societies.

REFERENCES

Aron, R. (1968). *Main Currents in Sociological Thought*. Vol. I. Garden City, NY: Anchor Books.

Blumer, H. (1969). *Symbolic Interactionism: Perspective and Method*. Englewood Cliffs, NJ: Prentice-Hall.

Bourdieu, P. (1992). *An Introduction to Reflexive Sociology*. Chicago: University of Chicago Press.

Bourdieu, P. (1993). *The Field of Cultural Production.* NY: Columbia University Press.

Caro, M.J., & Murphy, J.W. (2003). *El Mundo de la Cultura Cuántica.* Granada, Spain: Port Royal.

Choi, J.M., & Murphy, J.W. (1992). *The Politics and Philosophy of Political Correctness.* Westport, CT: Praeger.

Durkheim, E. (1984). *Pragmatism and Sociology.* Cambridge: Cambridge University Press.

Fish, S. (1989). *Doing What Comes Naturally.* Durham, NC: Duke University Press.

Garfinkel, H. (1967). *Studies in Ethnomethodology.* Englewood Cliffs, NJ: Prentice-Hall.

Gebser, J. (1985). *The Ever-Present Origin.* Athens, OH: Ohio University Press.

Lyotard, J.F. (1984). *The Postmodern Condition.* Minneapolis: University of Minnesota Press.

Morales, G. (1998). *El Cadáver de Balzac.* Alicante: Ediciones Epigono.

Murphy, J.W., & Caro, M.J. (2002). Alejandro Serrano y la Globalización desde Abajo. *Estudios Centroamericanos,* 647, 803-813.

Parsons, T. (1963). *The Social System.* Glencoe, IL: Glencoe Press.

Schlesinger, A.M. (1993). *The Disuniting of America.* NY: W.W. Norton and Company.

Conclusion

John W. Murphy
John T. Pardeck

During the 1960s, social interventions were expected to be enacted within the context supplied by the Community Mental Health Act of 1963 (Vega and Murphy, 1990). Services, in short, were supposed to be community-based. This phrase was interpreted to mean that persons should be treated in the least restrictive environment–which usually meant their communities–and be allowed to participate closely in the planning and execution of any intervention.

Following this general shift in orientation, a culture-based model of illness was adopted. Treatments, accordingly, should be sensitive to how persons define their problems and the types of interventions they believe are appropriate and effective. Additionally, treatment teams should no longer be dominated by medical specialists, but instead include a variety of perspectives. Physiological reductionism was thus replaced by a more expansive view of the nature of social problems.

This trend continued into the 1970s, although in a somewhat weakened form. For example, the medical establishment was somewhat reluctant to change and suffer a loss of prestige. Furthermore, insurance companies, because they controlled the purse strings, were slow to question the medical model. After all, when defined as physical illnesses, problems could be treated in an unambiguous manner. Nonethe-

[Haworth co-indexing entry note]: "Conclusion." Murphy, John W., and John T. Pardeck. Co-published simultaneously in *Journal of Social Work in Disability & Rehabilitation* (The Haworth Social Work Practice Press, an imprint of The Haworth Press, Inc.) Vol. 4, No. 1/2, 2005, pp. 165-169; and: *Disability Issues for Social Workers and Human Services Professionals in the Twenty-First Century* (ed: John W. Murphy, and John T. Pardeck) The Haworth Social Work Practice Press, an imprint of The Haworth Press, Inc., 2005, pp. 165-169. Single or multiple copies of this article are available for a fee from The Haworth Document Delivery Service [1-800-HAWORTH, 9:00 a.m. - 5:00 p.m. (EST). E-mail address: docdelivery@haworthpress.com].

http://www.haworthpress.com/web/JSWDR
Digital Object Identifier: 10.1300/J198v04n01_10

less, the memory of this landmark legislation was still fresh in the mind of most practitioners.

With the onset of the 1980s, and the ascendance of Reagan and Thatcher to power, the so-called Conservative Revolution was underway. In addition to politics, social service delivery was affected dramatically by this change. The medical model was again elevated in importance, with almost every behavior defined in physiological terms. For example, claims were made that perhaps crime and poverty might have genetic causes. And the growth of computer use, along with the proliferation of high-tech methodologies, reinforced the belief that interventions should become increasingly scientific (Murphy and Pardeck, 1991). Soon talk about holism and community sensitivity was envisioned to impede the creation of economically efficient interventions. Rather than activists, many practitioners became technicians and consultants.

This conservative backlash continues today. Although resistance is growing to the medicalization of clients, social problems are still portrayed regularly as personal issues that are tied intimately to biological causes. And instead of containing a modicum of institutional analysis and criticism, which conservatives are loath to consider, interventions focus mostly on the individual or the family.

In this regard, individualized therapies, along with drug treatment, are touted to enable troubled persons to cope better with the stress of everyday life. The idea that interventions might be designed to alter society is presumed to be a remnant of outmoded and ineffective utopianism. In effect, many practitioners have been convinced that they should be more pragmatic and lower their expectations. In many cases they have been intimidated by the current political climate.

THE PRESENT VOLUME

The papers contained in this volume suggest that interventions will have to change significantly in the coming years. Although in different ways, the authors contend that those with disabilities and other issues have been shortchanged by the clinical definitions that have been adopted during the past twenty years. Despite the existence of various protest movements, not to mention powerful legislation, reductionism prevails. With few exceptions, persons are evaluated mostly in terms of how far they deviate from the norm and their prospects for successful assimilation.

In a truly conservative manner, full citizenship depends on the ability and willingness to adjust to mainstream renditions of normalcy. Pluralism is thus eschewed, and those who demand to be recognized on their own terms are dismissed as incorrigible and making excessive demands. Those who dare to challenge the social or cultural *status quo*, and refuse to view themselves as deficient, continue to linger on the margins of society. Of course, remediation is offered, but the cost is often the dignity of those who are the focus of an intervention.

The authors of these papers advance several themes that may prove to be helpful in correcting this situation:

> A. A more holistic vision must be adopted, because today's society is replete with alienation. Persons have been convinced that they are objects and regularly treat one another in insensitive ways. Interventions should be designed, accordingly, that liberate persons from institutions that demand their self-effacement in order to be considered normal and useful (Martín-Baró, 1994). Support should be provided, accordingly, for them to engage in self-reflection and develop their unique capacities. Instead of trying to normalize persons, interventions should be constructed that address how they can create meaningful lives for themselves.

> B. Practitioners should reject the currently accepted strategies that medicalize clients. Although persons have a bodily presence, and problems are often manifested physically, physiology should not be mistaken as the source of all behavior. Such reductionism is misleading and ignores factors related to exploitation, racism, economic deprivation, and other considerations indicative of the misuse of power. Therefore, a range of vital social variables should be a part of any assessment of clients or interventions.

> C. All interventions should have a strong component of community involvement. Persons should be allowed to define their problems, identify appropriate remedies, construct therapies, and evaluate their progress. Most important is that communities must be provided with the training, funds, and other resources necessary for them to control their destinies. The decentralization of planning without the accompanying power does not necessarily improve the delivery of services.

D. In order for this involvement to occur, strident policy initiatives are required. Although the relevant legislation is often in place, and politicians are aware of their right to intervene, policy recommendations have been timid. Bold steps must be taken to eliminate all organizational, political, economic, and other barriers to the full inclusion of community members in the formulation and implementation of culturally sensitive interventions. Hence, unrelenting activism is required to address any institutional inequalities and traditions that stifle critique and unrestricted participation.

E. Central to this inclusiveness are issues related to diversity. Every effort must be made so that persons who were formerly marginalized are heard and treated equitably. Additionally, diverse intellectual styles, knowledge bases, cultural mores, and political positions must be given serious attention. A culture of democracy, in short, must be created whereby a full range of persons and viewpoints, even those that might be treated initially as utopian, can be given a fair hearing. In this sense, the philosophical and practical maneuvers must be made that reveal diversity to be an asset, rather than a liability to social existence. As a result, perhaps novel opinions and intervention strategies will begin to be recognized as viable.

FINAL THOUGHTS

Despite the rhetoric of various politicians, the social world is becoming an increasingly hostile place. In many respects persons are alienated, but have retained enough of their humanity to feel their loss. Consequently, almost on a daily basis, demands are heard for increased tranquility and community. The primary response, however, has been the distribution of more psychotropic drugs and other psychiatric palliatives.

But these responses blame the victims and place the burden of reform on these individuals. Those who suffer the most, accordingly, are often heard lamenting that their lives might have been different if only they had tried harder or made different choices. On the other hand, the culprit is not necessarily some abstract and faceless system. Using this sort of language does not help matters, and may in fact increase feelings of powerlessness. The critique that is needed nowadays must go beyond both of these elements and be more focused and progressive.

The medical system, for example, is not an impenetrable maze, but consists of concrete persons and policies that put profitability and political advantage ahead of health care for the masses. Certain politicians even want to prevent elderly persons from obtaining their medications from cheaper Canadian sources when they are available. The point, therefore, is this: the future should be spent unraveling and rethinking health care institutions, and the accompanying delivery systems, so that persons can control these entities and make them reflect their needs and priorities. These organizations, in other words, must no longer remain oligarchies, controlled by those who have little regard for well-being of the citizenry.

Such a change would mean that persons have control of their respective futures. They could define and support themselves, rather than be at the whim of so-called market, historical, or institutional forces. With a community of full participants, alienation and strife would not have to be thought of as natural or inevitable. And perhaps, finally, the enormous amount of resources that has been created by the general public could be put in the service of humanity, so that the better life that is possible might be realized by all persons.

REFERENCES

Martín-Baró, I. (1994). *Writing for a Liberation Psychology*. Cambridge, MA: Harvard University Press.

Murphy, J. W., & Pardeck, J. T. (1991). *The Computerization of Social Service Agencies*. Westport, CT: Auburn House.

Vega, W. A., & Murphy, J. W. (1990). *Culture and the Restructuring of Community Mental Health*. Westport, CT: Greenwood.

Index

BOOK ORDER FORM!

Order a copy of this book with this form or online at:
http://www.haworthpress.com/store/product.asp?sku=5445

Disability Issues for Social Workers and Human Services Professionals in the Twenty-First Century

_____ in softbound at $22.95 ISBN: 0-7890-2714-3.
_____ in hardbound at $ 34.95 ISBN: 0-7890-2713-5.

COST OF BOOKS _____

POSTAGE & HANDLING _____
US: $4.00 for first book & $1.50
for each additional book
Outside US: $5.00 for first book
& $2.00 for each additional book.

SUBTOTAL _____

In Canada: add 7% GST. _____

STATE TAX _____
CA, IL, IN, MN, NJ, NY, OH, PA & SD residents
please add appropriate local sales tax.

FINAL TOTAL _____
If paying in Canadian funds, convert
using the current exchange rate,
UNESCO coupons welcome.

❑ BILL ME LATER:
Bill-me option is good on US/Canada/
Mexico orders only; not good to jobbers,
wholesalers, or subscription agencies.

❑ Signature _____

❑ Payment Enclosed: $ _____

❑ PLEASE CHARGE TO MY CREDIT CARD:
❑ Visa ❑ MasterCard ❑ AmEx ❑ Discover
❑ Diner's Club ❑ Eurocard ❑ JCB

Account # _____

Exp Date _____

Signature _____
(Prices in US dollars and subject to change without notice.)

PLEASE PRINT ALL INFORMATION OR ATTACH YOUR BUSINESS CARD

Name

Address

City   State/Province   Zip/Postal Code

Country

Tel   Fax

E-Mail

May we use your e-mail address for confirmations and other types of information? ❑ Yes ❑ No We appreciate receiving
your e-mail address. Haworth would like to e-mail special discount offers to you, as a preferred customer.
We will never share, rent, or exchange your e-mail address. We regard such actions as an invasion of your privacy.

Order from your **local bookstore** or directly from
The Haworth Press, Inc. 10 Alice Street, Binghamton, New York 13904-1580 • USA
Call our toll-free number (1-800-429-6784) / Outside US/Canada: (607) 722-5857
Fax: 1-800-895-0582 / Outside US/Canada: (607) 771-0012
E-mail your order to us: orders@haworthpress.com

For orders outside US and Canada, you may wish to order
through your local
sales representative, distributor, or bookseller.
For information, see http://haworthpress.com/distributors

(Discounts are available for individual orders in US and Canada only, not booksellers/distributors.)
Please photocopy this form for your personal use.
www.HaworthPress.com

BOF05